W9-BCD-047

Library Services

for Disabled Individuals

WITHDRAWN
NDSU

Library Services
for Disabled Individuals

RASHELLE S. KARP

G.K. Hall & Co.
Boston, Massachusetts

All rights reserved.
Copyright 1991 G.K. Hall.

First published 1991
by G.K. Hall & Co.
70 Lincoln Street
Boston, Massachusetts 02111

10 9 8 7 6 5 4 3 2 1

Library of Congress Cataloging-in-Publication Data

Library services for disabled individuals / [compiled by] Rashelle S.
Karp.
    p. cm.
    Includes bibliographical references and index.
    ISBN 0-8161-1927-9 – ISBN 0-8161-1928-7 (pbk.)
    1. Libraries and the handicapped. 2. Handicapped – Services for.
I. Karp, Rashelle S.
  Z711.92.H3L518   1991
  027.6'63 – dc20   91-10996
                                            CIP

The paper used in this publication meets the minimum requirements of
American National Standard for Information Sciences – Permanence of
Paper for Printed Library Materials. ANSI Z39.48-1984.   ∞™
MANUFACTURED IN THE UNITED STATES OF AMERICA

Contents

Preface

This book has been designed to provide the information and supplementary material necessary for a librarian to feel comfortable with his or her knowledge about the needs of and appropriate library services for disabled patrons. It may also be used as the basis for conducting an in-service workshop on library services for disabled patrons. There are four informational chapters, each of which deals with a different type of disability (learning disability, blindness and/or visual impairment, deafness and/or hearing impairment, and mental retardation). Topics covered in these chapters include legislation that mandates or facilitates service; the demographics, characteristics, and library and information needs of library patrons with a specific disability; the services, programs, or resources librarians can offer to facilitate access for patrons with a specific disability; and a selective list of agencies that can provide information and help. An appendix contains simple exercises that will sensitize librarians to the needs and difficulties of disabled library patrons, and an annotated bibliography provides sources for further reading on library services to the disabled.

Intended for public, school, academic, and special librarians, as well as for library school students, *Library Services for Disabled Individuals* has been prepared by professionals in the field. The information provided has been selected for its practical and reference value.

Library Services to Individuals with Learning Disabilities

RASHELLE S. KARP

Associate Professor of Library Science
Clarion University of Pennsylvania

Definitions and Federal Legislation

Federal legislation relating to learning disabilities revolves around definitions of the term as it applies to children and their education. Because of this, the legislation and definitions of learning disabilities are covered in the same section of this chapter.

The Education of All Handicapped Children Act of 1975 (PL 94-142) first referred to learning disabilities as a group of disabilities requiring educational remediation. The term was defined in 1977, when the U.S. Office of Education released the following definition:

> "Specific learning disability" means a disorder in one or more of the basic psychological processes involved in understanding or in using language, spoken or written, which may manifest itself in an imperfect ability to listen, think, speak, read, write, spell, or to do mathematical calculations. The term includes such conditions as perceptual handicaps, brain injury, minimal brain dysfunction, dyslexia, and developmental aphasia. The term does not include children who have learning problems which are primarily the result of visual, hearing, or motor handicaps, of mental

retardation, or emotional disturbance, or of environmental, cultural, or economic disadvantage (U.S. Office of Education, 1977, p. 65083).

Within this definition, three significant criteria are presented that help educators identify learning disabled children. First, learning disabled children must exhibit a severe discrepancy between their achievement and their intellectual ability, or they must not be performing commensurate with their age and ability levels when provided learning experiences appropriate for their age and ability level. Second, this discrepancy cannot be primarily the result of a visual, motor, or hearing handicap; mental retardation; emotional disturbance; or environmental, cultural, or economic disadvantage. Third, learning disabilities affect a person's abilities in one or more of the following areas: oral expression, listening comprehension, written expression, basic reading skills, reading comprehension, mathematics calculation, or mathematics reasoning.

A fourth concept that is mentioned, but not explicated, in the 1977 definition is that of perceptual handicaps. These have been defined by practitioners as the inability to recognize, discriminate, and interpret stimuli, especially visual, auditory, and tactile stimuli.

In 1988, the National Joint Committee for Learning Disabilities (NJCLD) agreed upon a definition of learning disabilities that recognized their existence in adults, as well as in children:

> *Learning disabilities* is a generic term that refers to a heterogeneous group of disorders manifested by significant difficulties in the acquisition and use of listening, speaking, reading, writing, reasoning, or mathematical abilities. These disorders are intrinsic to the individual, presumed to be due to central nervous system dysfunction, and may occur across the life span. Problems in self-regulatory behaviors, social perception, and social interaction may exist with learning disabilities, but do not by themselves constitute a learning disability. Although learning disabilities may occur concomitantly with other handicapping conditions (for example, sensory impairment, mental retardation, social and emotional disturbance) or with extrinsic influences (such as cultural differences, insufficient or inappropriate instruction), they are not the result of those conditions or influences (NJCLD, 1988, p. 1).

Both definitions stress that learning disabilities may occur with other disabilities but that they are not the result of other disabilities. This means, for example, that learning disabilities are not the same as mental retardation. In fact, learning disabled children must, if they are to be identified as primarily learning disabled, have average or above average IQs.

Many professionals and professional associations have augmented or opposed these definitions. (For a more detailed discussion, see the Hammill, 1990 reference in the bibliography.) The legal definition stands, however. It, along with the NJCLD expansion, is used for this chapter.

Characteristics of Learning Disabilities

Learning disabilities are a complex and confusing group of impairments that may manifest themselves as academic problems, language disorders, perceptual disorders, metacognitive deficits, social and emotional problems, motor disorders, and attention problems. To varying degrees, individuals with learning disabilities will have problems in one or more of the areas listed below.

Reading Skills. Reading skills may be characterized by dyslexia. This means that a learning disabled person's reading will suffer from poor decoding and word recognition skills, resulting in slow reading and, often, incomplete understanding of the meaning conveyed by the words being read.

Writing Skills and Written Expression. Writing and written expression may be characterized by dysgraphia. This means that a learning disabled person's handwriting may suffer from illegibility, poor slant and formation of letters, cramping of letters, and a lack of flow from letter to letter. Organization of thoughts will often be poor, when they must be written down, and written vocabulary may be much lower than oral vocabulary. Finally, written expression may be characterized by many cross-outs and erasures, which indicate difficulty writing rather than just the normal editing process.

Spelling. Spelling errors may be excessive and phonetically inaccurate. Spelling may also be characterized by reversals of letters, omissions or additions of letters, and arbitrary repetition of letters. Often, words beginning with vowels are difficult to spell, and vowel confusion is evident in the spelling of other words.

Arithmetic and Mathematical Reasoning. The ability to do arithmetic and to use mathematical reasoning may be characterized by dyscalculia. This means that learning disabled persons may have problems performing tasks involved in mathematical calculations. They may also have problems conceptualizing mathematical abstractions and applying mathematical concepts.

Memory and Thinking. A learning disabled individual may have poor ability in abstract reasoning, resulting in poor cognitive sequencing (thinking in an orderly way) and poor cognitive discrimination (distinguishing between two similar concepts). Depending upon how the learning disability manifests itself, a learning disabled person may exhibit poor short term or poor long term memory. Some learning disabled individuals also suffer from agnosia, or the inability to recognize familiar objects through the use of the senses.

Intelligence. Learning disabled individuals must have IQs that are average or above average. An individual with an IQ score lower than 65-75 is no longer considered learning disabled but rather is considered mentally retarded. It cannot be stressed enough: Although a mentally retarded individual may also have specific learning disabilities, an individual who is identified as only learning disabled will possess average or above average intelligence. It should also be noted that the diagnostic procedures for identifying individuals with learning disabilities often begin by identifying individuals whose scores on a traditional IQ test are below average. Further testing that measures specific abilities will reveal test scores that are not low all the way across but, rather, are low only in the areas in which a learning disability is present.

Activity Level and Attention Span. Individuals who are learning disabled may exhibit signs of either hyperactivity or hypoactivity. They may also suffer from short attention spans or may be easily distracted by stimuli in their environment. They may also have impaired selective attention, resulting in problems (1) selecting relevant material from irrelevant or background material and (2) maintaining attention to relevant material. On the other end, the attention of some learning disabled individuals may be characterized by perseveration, or fixed attentiveness to a single task, motor activity, or verbal topic that is repeated over and over. Problems with attention can impair the ability to make decisions, especially from many choices, and to organize experience.

Motor Coordination. Sometimes an individual's learning disability is characterized by poor gross motor coordination, poor fine motor coordination, or both. Poor gross motor coordination manifests itself in poor balance, awkwardness, and clumsiness; poor fine motor coordination manifests itself in poor handwriting, difficulties typing, and difficulties with other tasks that require good hand to eye coordination.

Tactual Perception. Some learning disabled individuals may have difficulty with touch because they suffer from an imperfect ability to interpret tactual stimuli. For example, they may have a need to touch objects to adequately interpret them, or, conversely, they may avoid touching and being touched because they cannot accurately perceive the pressure that is being applied.

Proxemic Perception. Characteristic of some learning disabled individuals is an imperfect awareness of the relationship among parts of their own bodies. They may also be imperfectly aware of their body's orientation, position, and movement in space and time. These types of problems may cause learning disabled individuals to be late for appointments, to stand too close to someone while talking with them, to confuse left with right, or to have difficulties reading a map or directional signs.

Auditory/Visual Motor Coordination. Learning disabled individuals with auditory motor problems will have difficulty copying something they have only heard (i.e., taking notes from an oral lecture, dancing to a rhythmic sound, following verbal directions). Visual motor problems cause difficulties copying something a learning disabled person has only seen (i.e., copying written instructions, copying telephone numbers off of a television screen, learning a dance step that has been demonstrated visually).

Auditory/Visual Discrimination. Often, learning disabled individuals will experience difficulty distinguishing between similar visual stimuli (i.e., the difference between *e* and *c*, or the difference between two shades of the same color) or between similar auditory stimuli (i.e., the difference between *th* and *f*, *17* and *70*, or an angry tone of voice and a joking tone of voice).

Auditory/Visual Figure-Ground. The inability to attend to important visual or auditory stimuli in the presence of background stimuli is sometimes a characteristic of learning disabled people. For example, learning disabled individuals may not find a specific person in a crowd or may not be able to read one line of print on a full page of print. They may not be able to hear a telephone ringing over music in the background, or they may not be able to hear talking over party noises.

Auditory/Visual Closure and Sequencing. Learning disabled individuals may have difficulty filling in missing parts of an incomplete word, sentence, or thought (closure). Having trouble seeing or hearing things in their correct order (sequencing) is also common among learning disabled individuals. For example, they may see words or letters reversed, cans on a grocery shelf reversed, or books on a library shelf reversed. They may hear the word *treats* instead of the word *street*, or music may sound garbled to them because the notes are out of order.

Auditory/Visual Memory. Some learning disabled individuals will experience problems remembering or revisualizing images or sequences that were originally presented to them visually. For example, they may have difficulty remembering a story or a passage in a book. Conversely, some learning disabled individuals may have trouble remembering or repeating concepts or sequences that were originally presented to them orally. For example, they may have difficulty remembering a story that was read aloud or directions that were given orally.

Receptive Language. Sometimes learning disabled individuals experience difficulty gaining meaning from spoken or written language. This difficulty may be caused by some of the problems explained above, or it may be caused by the slowed speed at which some learning disabled people decode written and spoken language. It is estimated, for example, that to understand a written passage, a person must read at least 175 to 300 words

5

per minute. Learning disabled individuals with dyslexia might be able to read a passage, but the rate at which they read might be too slow to understand the concepts presented.

Central or Inner Language. While some learning disabled individuals have problems gaining meaning from spoken or written language, some also have problems organizing the thought processes used to communicate within themselves. This can cause delayed responses to communications from others and delayed initiation of communication to others.

Expressive Language. Problems of organization can affect learning disabled persons' capacity for self-expression. For example, a person may have difficulty organizing and producing phrases, clauses, or sentences. Preoccupation with the process of constructing a sentence may mean that not enough attention is paid to the medium through which the sentence is relayed. For example, a learning disabled person's speech may be toneless and slow, or it could be marked with speech irregularities (e.g., run-on sentences or short sentences).

Work Habits. Because of the problems that many learning disabled individuals experience with reading and writing, they may work more slowly than employers expect.

Social/Emotional Behavior. Learning disabled people are *not* socially or emotionally disturbed. Their actions, however, may sometimes be characterized by impulsiveness and by failure to think carefully about the consequences of certain behaviors. They may exhibit poor group relationships or poor judgment in social and interpersonal relationships. This may be in part because they are working so hard to understand the words of peers that they may miss the nonverbal cues. Missing nonverbal cues can also cause behavior that is usually considered inappropriate (i.e., lack of tact, lack of awareness of their impact on others). Often, learning disabled individuals are field dependent; that is, they are not self-sufficient. Their self-esteem comes from what others think of them, and they are likely to conform to peer pressure.

Metacognition. Sometimes learning disabled individuals experience metacognitive deficits, or dysfunctions in the ways they learn. An inability to "learn how to learn" can severely hinder a learning disabled person's analysis and synthesis of new knowledge. The field of metacognition is relatively new, but some researchers are enjoying success in their attempts to teach learning strategies to learning disabled individuals with metacognitive deficits (Deschler, Warner, Schumaker, and Alley, 1983).

Intersensory Mechanisms. Some learning disabled individuals will have difficulty using two senses at once. For example, they may not feel a tap on the shoulder while they are absorbed in a television program or a book.

It must be emphasized that not all of these deficits will occur at the same time. A learning disabled individual will exhibit one or more of these problems.

Universal Needs of Learning Disabled Individuals and How They Translate into Library Services

To varying degrees, depending upon the severity and areas of impact, learning disabled individuals may require special attention in the library, including the following areas.

Need for Directional Assistance. Because of the problems that some learning disabled individuals may have with the physical application of directions, many will require individualized help, reinforced by repetition. In a library, individualized help may be necessary to facilitate:

1. Orientation to the building. Clear and repeated signage to all possible destinations is very helpful.

2. Orientation to the location of specific library staff members. Again, clear and repeated signs to service points are very helpful. Also, identifying badges (i.e., reference staff) can help direct learning disabled patrons as well as all other patrons to appropriate service points.

3. Orientation to specific stack areas. As before, clear and repeated signs, especially signs on each bay of shelving, are very helpful. It is also helpful to shelve materials in the same physical order (i.e., left to right or right to left) throughout the library. If the library is on more than one floor, each floor should be clearly labeled; the items each floor contains should also be clearly labeled.

4. Orientation and reinforcement of the library's classification system. Learning disabled patrons with directional problems may not have difficulties finding desired items in the library's catalog. However, getting to the shelves and then selecting the specific item may be problematic. The clear signage mentioned before can reduce problems with locating general shelving areas, and a consistent physical order for shelving is also helpful. A librarian or staff person may still need to help a learning disabled individual translate the abstract number written on the card to a physical location on a shelf full of books. The need for this type of assistance may lessen as the patron becomes more practiced. In some cases, assistance may always be necessary. It is important to note that the concepts

involved in understanding classification are not necessarily the problem; the problem is the inability of some learning disabled individuals to apply an abstract direction to a concrete physical location.

Need for Reading Assistance. Because of visual processing deficits, many learning disabled patrons experience reading difficulties. One of the most effective ways for librarians to provide reading assistance is through the provision of high interest/low vocabulary materials. By using less complex literary structures, hi/low reading materials allow learning disabled patrons to read about topics at all levels of interest and intellectual capacity. Sometimes the device of putting less print on a page is all that is needed to facilitate reading by a person who suffers from dyslexia. Sometimes less complex vocabulary and simpler sentence structures are necessary. The variability of needs in this area requires that librarians not only add specifically designed hi/low materials to library collections but also examine their existing collections to determine if items already in the collection might satisfy some hi/low needs. Some criteria, in addition to those generally used to select materials, are helpful to apply.

1. Does the context of a sentence give clues about the meaning of more difficult words?

2. Is information presented in its simplest or most direct written form?

3. Are there illustrations, chapter headings, marginal notes, or other devices that organize the material?

4. Is there enough white space on the pages to eliminate crowding of letters?

5. Is the print size large enough to facilitate visual discrimination between letters, words, and paragraphs?

6. Is the paper opaque (to avoid confusing "see through" from the other side)?

7. For fiction, is the story line so complex that it requires tremendous memory or great organizational skills?

It is important to note that not all of these criteria need to be met for each selected item. Depending upon the type of learning disability, even one accommodation (i.e., more white space on the page) might make the difference between reading or not reading. The American Library

Association, the National Council of Teachers of English, the International Reading Association, and other agencies and publishers often produce lists of reading materials that are specifically in the hi/low format, or that qualify as hi/low even though not specifically written in that form. Some recent resources are the National Council of Teachers of English (1988) *High Interest Easy Reading*, the International Reading Association's (1989) *Easy Reading*, Gale Research Company's *High Interest Books for Teens* (1988), and LiBretto's *High-Low Handbook* (Bowker, 1990). Librarians also should not forget to examine resources that list materials appropriate for adult new readers.

Need for Elimination of Architectural Barriers. Learning disabled individuals who are affected in the area of gross motor coordination will benefit greatly from architectural modifications that provide unimpeded access to all areas of the library.

Need for Elimination of Distractions. Learning disabled individuals with attention deficits may require quiet areas that will facilitate their concentration (i.e., library carrels).

Need for Materials that Aid Development of Motor Skills. Toys, games, and puzzles can help learning disabled children who have difficulties in the area of motor skills.

Need for Information about Learning Disabilities. Because learning disabilities are so complex and difficult to diagnose, it is especially important that library collections provide information about learning disabilities, both for learning disabled individuals and for their families and friends. Information on diagnosis, remediation, coping skills, and local, state, and national agencies from which help can be received should be made available. The information should be provided at appropriate reading levels.

Need for Early Identification and Aggressive Intervention. A key to helping someone compensate for a learning disability lies in early identification, which allows remediation to occur before, rather than after, problems develop. For example, a child with dyslexia could begin learning compensation techniques before reading instruction begins in the schools. Not only early identification is important; so is aggressive intervention. Learning disabled individuals are often shy and are sometimes reluctant to ask questions. The techniques that a reference librarian uses to initiate and develop communication with all shy patrons should be aggressively used with shy learning disabled patrons.

Need for Alternative Formats of Information. Learning disabled individuals can often benefit from nontraditional formats of information. Most helpful are recordings that can be used in conjunction with the printed sources from which they were made. Listening to the words as they follow along on the printed page can develop learning disabled individuals' sight vocabulary, increase comprehension because two modalities (visual and

9

auditory) are used at the same time, decrease the frustration often felt when reading, and provide successful experiences with reading.

Especially helpful for learning disabled individuals with reading problems are the services provided by the Library of Congress's National Library Service for the Blind and Physically Handicapped. Children and adults whose learning disabilities are certified by a medical doctor qualify for the provision of recorded materials (tape and record), free of charge, from the National Library Service. Librarians should maintain and disseminate application forms for these services. (Application forms can be obtained from the Library of Congress or from one of the regional libraries located throughout the country.) The materials provided by the National Library Service primarily consist of leisure reading (fiction and nonfiction) and magazines in recorded format. Individuals who qualify for service from the National Library Service also qualify for service from Recording for the Blind, which provides textbooks in recorded format. Both services provide recorded materials on a loan basis, but loan periods can, in some cases, be as long as a year or more. Since neither of these services provides print copies of the books it records, local collections of print materials that parallel the recorded materials borrowed by learning disabled individuals can be very helpful.

Need for Immediate Feedback to Help Maintain Motivation. A commonly used technique for providing immediate and continuous feedback is computer-assisted instruction (CAI). Because the computer is dedicated only to its immediate user, it, unlike group instruction, can deliver immediate, continuous, and differentiated responses to the individual using it. Much software has been developed that focuses on either remediation or the development of compensation techniques for learning disabled individuals. Software designed to teach learning disabled students is available at reasonable cost and can be added to a library's circulating collection, or, if the library has public access microcomputers, the packages can be added to a reference collection. Like all materials, there are good and bad software packages. Preview is strongly recommended, and consistent application of selection criteria is paramount. The American Library Association has published a particularly useful resource that provides criteria for evaluating educational software (see Doll, 1987, resource in the bibliography).

Need to Experience Success. Learning disabled individuals often experience failure, especially academic failure and especially if their learning disabilities are not identified early. The most effective way to combat experiences of failure is to provide experiences of success. Because libraries are noncompetitive and librarians are typically not involved in evaluation of patron performance, they are ideal facilitators of success. Merely by continuing to apply the most basic principles of librarianship – "Every reader, his book; every book, its reader" (Ranganathan, cited in Gopinath,

1978) – librarians can provide a plethora of successful, esteem-building experiences for learning disabled patrons.

Need for Individualized Interactions to Supplement Mass Media Communications. Often, learning disabled individuals require individualized instruction or explanation of information presented in group situations. Librarianship is based in large part upon such individualized interactions. Reference services, bibliographic instruction, reader's advisory, and information and referral services rely upon individually tailored communication and can be excellent complements to large group communications.

Need to Feel in Control of Tasks and Outcomes Assessment. Feelings of empowerment are important to everyone, but they are especially helpful for learning disabled individuals, who, because of their disability, may feel that their disability controls them. Contract learning, where students are responsible for determining the pace and scope of a learning project as well as the way they will evaluate their success, has been used successfully with learning disabled students in the schools. Library services are in some ways very similar to contract learning in that patrons determine the pace and scope of their reading, the evaluation of their success, and even the success of the reading material. The feelings of control that frequent use of the library can foster are invaluable to individuals who may not feel totally in control anywhere else.

Agencies That Can Provide Information and Help

Association for Children and Adults with Learning Disabilities
4156 Library Road
Pittsburgh, PA 15234

Comprised of parents of children with learning disabilities and professionals in the field, the association disseminates information and provides assistance to state and local groups. It publishes *Learning Disabilities*.

Association of Learning Disabled Adults
PO Box 9722, Friendship Station
Washington, DC 20016

This self-help network of adults (learning disabled and not disabled), institutions, and agencies focuses on developing coping skills for adults with learning disabilities by sponsoring discussion groups, a speakers' bureau, and social activities.

Council for Learning Disabilities
PO Box 40303
Overland Park, KS 66204

Comprised of professionals in the area of learning disabilities, the council works to improve education of learning disabled individuals by improving teacher preparation programs as well as local educational programs. The council publishes *LD Forum* and *Learning Disability Quarterly*.

Council for Exceptional Children
Division for Learning Disabilities
1920 Association Drive
Reston, VA 22091

The council provides computer searches and citations from professional materials related to the education of handicapped and gifted young people.

National Center for Learning Disabilities
99 Park Ave., 6th Floor
New York, NY 10016

This volunteer organization promotes public awareness of the problems of learning disabilities by making available resources, providing referrals to professionals, conducting seminars, and funding innovative programs in the field of learning disabilities. It has funded public library programs.

National Library Service for the Blind and Physically Handicapped
Library of Congress
1291 Taylor Street, NW
Washington, DC 20542

The National Library Service provides recorded materials (tape and record) and braille materials for individuals who are visually impaired, physically disabled, or learning disabled (medically certified).

National Network of Learning Disabled Adults
808 N. 82d Street, Suite F2
Scottsdale, AZ 85257

The network disseminates information about learning disabilities to its members, maintains a speakers' bureau, sponsors competitions, compiles statistics, and bestows awards in the field. The network maintains an electronic bulletin board called *LD Adult*.

Orton Dyslexia Society
724 York Road
Baltimore, MD 21204

The society is an excellent source of information about dyslexia. It publishes *Annals of Dyslexia*.

Recording for the Blind
20 Roszel Road
Princeton, NJ 08540

Recording for the Blind is a major source of recorded textbooks for visually impaired persons and persons with medically certified learning disabilities.

References

Deschler, D. D., M. M. Warner, J. B. Schumaker, and G. R. Alley. 1983. "Learning Strategies Intervention Model." In *Current Topics in Learning Disabilities*, edited by J. D. McKinney and L. Feagans, 245-84. Norwood, N.J.: Ablex.

Doll, C. A. 1987. *Evaluating Educational Software*. Chicago: American Library Association.

Gopinath, M. A. 1978. "Ranganathan." In *Encyclopedia of Library and Information Science*, edited by A. Kent, H. Lancour, and J. E. Daily. New York: Marcel Dekker.

Hammill, D. D. 1990. "On Defining Learning Disabilities: An Emerging Consensus." *Journal of Learning Disabilities* 23, no. 2 (February): 74-85.

LiBretto, E. V. 1990. *High-Low Handbook: Books, Materials, and Services for the Problem Reader*. New York: Bowker.

Matthews, D. 1988. *High Interest Easy Reading*. Urbana, Ill.: National Council of Teachers of English.

Nakamura, J. 1988. *High Interest Books For Teens*. Detroit, Mich.: Gale Research Company.

National Joint Committee on Learning Disabilities. 1988. Letter to NJCLD member organizations quoted in Hammill, "On Defining Learning Disabilities."

R. J. Ryder, B. B. Graves, and M. F. Graves. 1989. *Easy Reading: Book Series and Periodicals for Less Able Readers*. Newark, Del.: International Reading Association.

U.S. Office of Education. 1977. "Assistance to States for Education of Handicapped Children: Procedures for Evaluating Specific Learning Disabilities." *Federal Register* 42: 65082-85.

Library Services to Mentally Retarded Individuals

PAMELA GENT

Assistant Professor of Special Education
Clarion University of Pennsylvania

Definitions

The most widely accepted definition of mental retardation comes from the American Association for Mental Retardation (AAMR), which defines mental retardation as "significantly subaverage general intellectual functioning existing concurrently with deficits in adaptive behavior and manifested during the development period" (Grossman, 1983, p. 11).

Significantly subaverage general intellectual functioning translates into low intelligence. What is intelligence, and how low must it be before it is significantly subaverage? Intelligence, unfortunately, is a nebulous and rather ill defined construct that, for the past century has been debated by scientists and researchers. The problem is that "No one . . . has seen a thing called intelligence. Rather, we observe differences in the way people behave" (Salvia and Ysseldyke, 1988, p. 147).

Psychologists and psychometricians who examine the behavior of individuals in specific testing situations measure intelligence through the use of intelligence tests. It is assumed that the scores on tests of intelligence actually represent intelligence and that individuals whose scores are high on intelligence tests are brighter than individuals whose scores are low. The most widely used tests of intelligence are the three Wechsler Scales (WISC-R, WAIS-R, WPPSI) (Wechsler, 1967; 1974; 1981) and the Stanford Binet Test (Thorndike, Hagen, and Sattler, 1986). On these tests and on other similar tests, a score from 0 to approximately 200 can be obtained. The scores are often called IQ (Intelligence Quotient) scores, and the average IQ score is 100. Figure 1 presents a graph of IQ normal distribution.

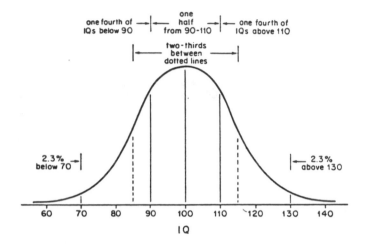

Figure 1. The "normal" distribution of IQs. This assumes a standard deviation of 15 points, characteristics of many scales. The Stanford-Binet has a standard deviation of 16 points; other scales have higher or lower values. By convention the mean IQ is always 100. The proportional values have been rounded.

H. J. Grossman, 1983. *Classification in Mental Retardation* (Washington, D.C.: American Association on Mental Deficiency), 31. Reprinted with permission of the American Association on Mental Deficiency.

As described by AAMR, persons who have significantly subaverage general intelligence have IQs of 70, plus or minus 5. The 10-point spread allows professionals a standard error of measure to compensate for variance of a person's score on an intelligence test as a result of chance.

The AAMR definition also mentions deficits in adaptive behavior. Adaptive behavior can be thought of as the degree to which a person meets his or her obligations, gets along in society, or is independent. The AAMR definition views adaptive behavior as the effectiveness with which one meets "the standards of personal independence, and/or social responsibility that are expected for his or her age level and cultural group" (Grossman, 1983, p. 11).

It follows that adaptive behavior cannot be measured in isolation but must be determined in relation to the age of the person and to the sociocultural group within which the person functions. Individuals with impairments in adaptive behavior would have difficulty conforming to and fulfilling the roles that their particular society has established for them (Salvia and Ysseldyke, 1988).

Impaired adaptive behavior is usually ascertained by interviewing a person who is very familiar with the individual who may be retarded. A psychologist or psychometrician asks the interviewee a structured series of questions designed to assess the presence of typical and atypical behavior.

The Vineland Adaptive Behavior Scale (Sparrow, Balla, and Cicchetti, 1984) and the American Association on Mental Deficiency (AAMD) Adaptive Behavior Scale for Children and Adults (Nihira, Foster, Shellhass, and Leland, 1974) are the most commonly used instruments to assess adaptive behavior.

Finally, the AAMR definition mentions the developmental period. What that encompasses has been widely discussed. (See Patton, Beirne-Smith, and Payne, 1990, for a more thorough discussion.) The AAMR now defines it as the period from conception to the 18th birthday (Grossman, 1983).

It is important to note that all three criteria – low intelligence, deficits in adaptive behavior, and manifestation of both during the developmental period – must be met prior to labeling a person mentally retarded. None of the three criteria alone is sufficient, nor is any combination of just two. As a case in point, one can consider the person who has an IQ of 65 and impairments in adaptive behavior as a result of injuries sustained in an automobile accident at age 27. Such a person would not be labeled mentally retarded because the low IQ and problems in adaptive behavior were not obvious until the 27th year. This person instead would be labeled head injured or developmentally disabled because all three criteria for mental retardation were not met.

The AAMR definition of mental retardation is the most widely accepted definition, but it is not the only one. Many states have developed their own definitions of mental retardation, which are similar but not identical to the AAMR definition. Frankenberger and Harper (1988) surveyed all 50 states and found that 86 percent of the states included measures of adaptive behavior in their definition of mental retardation. Some researchers (Hawkins and Cooper, 1990; Polloway and Smith, 1987) have found, however, that although the majority of the states reported that they consider adaptive behavior when making a determination of retardation, in actuality IQ is the sole criterion used. In other words, if the person meets the IQ criterion, it is automatically assumed that the person will meet the adaptive behavior criterion. It should also be noted that the IQ criterion in many states differs from that of the AAMR. A late 1980 survey found that 59

17

percent of the states used intelligence cutoff scores of 70 or 75 and 12.2 percent of the states specified intelligence cutoff scores of higher than 75. Remarkably, 26.8 percent of the states did not specify an intelligence test cutoff score (Frankenberger and Harper, 1988).

With a range of diagnostic IQ scores for people who are retarded from 0 to 70/75, considerable variability in terms of potential achievement is possible. Professionals, therefore, have found it useful to further delineate the population of individuals labeled mentally retarded into smaller groups. The AAMR definition categorizes mental retardation into four groups: mild, moderate, severe, and profound. Figure 2 graphically displays the categorization.

Figure 2. IQ Range and Level of Retardation

Level of Retardation	IQ Range
Mild	50/55 to 70/75
Moderate	35/40 to 50/55
Severe	20/25 to 35/40
Profound	Below 20/25

As may be seen in Figure 2, individuals labeled mildly retarded manifest IQs between 50/55 and 70/75, those labeled moderately retarded show IQs between 35/40 and 50/55, those labeled severely retarded manifest IQs between 20/25 and 35/40, and those labeled profoundly retarded show IQs lower than 20/25. The overlap between categories allows professionals to differentially label individuals who have similar IQ scores but great discrepancies in adaptive behavior. Consider, for example, two individuals with identical IQ scores of 55. One of these individuals has slight impairments in adaptive behavior; the other has none. The overlap permits a professional to label the person with no adaptive behavior impairments mildly retarded and the person with some impairments in adaptive behavior moderately retarded.

Some educational institutions have chosen to use different terms to describe the levels of retardation defined in Figure 2. Thus, the term *educable mentally retarded* (EMR) generally corresponds to the AAMR mildly retarded category, *trainable mentally retarded* (TMR) to the AAMR moderately retarded category, and *severely/profoundly mentally retarded* (SPMR) to the AAMR severely and profoundly retarded categories. Persons who are labeled mildly retarded or EMR comprise approximately 90 percent of all mentally retarded individuals, individuals who are moderately retarded or TMR make up 7 to 8 percent, and individuals labeled SPMR take up the remaining 2 to 3 percent.

EMR, TMR, and SPMR were originally coined to identify the type of school program in which students with mental retardation would be enrolled. For instance, students labeled EMR were placed in programs that emphasized reading, students labeled TMR were placed in programs that emphasized training in daily living skills, and students labeled SPMR were placed in programs that provided mere custodial care. Today, the definitions are used loosely, and professionals no longer base a student's educational program solely on these labels.

Demographics

When one attempts to determine how many persons are labeled mentally retarded, one immediately notes significant discrepancies, depending upon the source of the statistics. Using a purely statistical model based on the normal or Gaussian curve, one would estimate that 2.3 percent of the population would be labeled mentally retarded. Some (Grossman, 1983) report that 3 percent of the population is mentally retarded. Still others, including the U.S. government, report that 1 percent is mentally retarded (Broman, Nichols, Shaughnessy, and Kennedy, 1987; 11th Annual Report to Congress, 1989). The figures also vary widely from state to state. For example, Alaska reports that only 0.33 percent of the school population is mentally retarded, while Alabama reports that 3.32 percent of the population is mentally retarded. Most researchers now generally concur that approximately 1 percent of the population is mentally retarded, the bulk of whom are EMR, or mildly retarded.

Interestingly, the population of individuals who are labeled mentally retarded has declined significantly in the past decade. The U.S. government reported a 42 percent decrease in the number of school age students identified as mentally retarded from school year 1975-76 to 1987-88 (11th Annual Report to Congress, 1989). These decreases occurred mostly in the groups of students labeled EMR or mildly retarded (Frankenberger and Harper, 1988). Several reasons can account for this decline.

1. The definition of mental retardation has changed in two significant ways. In 1961, the score below which a person was considered mentally retarded was 80 (Heber, 1961). This allowed a potential 16 percent of the population to meet the criterion for mental retardation (Patton, Beirne-Smith, and Payne, 1990). In the past decade, however, the general score below which a person is considered mentally retarded has been lowered to a range of 65 to 75, thus greatly decreasing the number of individuals who test at a mental retardation level.

2. The definition of mental retardation has been changed to include an assessment of adaptive behavior. This has eliminated individuals who had come to be known as the "six hour retarded children" (President's Committee on Mental Retardation, 1970). These are children who had difficulty during the six-hour school day but who functioned normally in all other aspects of their lives. Although these children tested with low IQs, they had no deficits in adaptive behavior. A high score on an adaptive behavior test has, over the past decade, excluded these children from being labeled mentally retarded. The addition of adaptive behavior requirements has also allowed professionals to sort out individuals who are simply poor students from those who are truly retarded, resulting in a decline in the numbers of students labeled mildly mentally retarded.

3. Several court cases, most notably *Larry P. v. Riles* (1979), cited a larger percentage of minority students enrolled in special education classrooms than in the school district at large. For example, in the San Francisco Unified School District, the site of the *Larry P. v. Riles* case, the percentage of African-American students in special education classes was 25 percent, while the percentage of African-American students in the school population at large was 10 percent (Reschly, 1988). Parents and professionals speculated that the intelligence tests were biased against those from nonwhite cultural backgrounds. In the *Larry P. v. Riles* case, the courts concurred and ordered close examination of the tests used and the placement process used to place individuals into special education. As a result of this case and similar cases, school districts are now much more careful when labeling someone mentally retarded, which has caused a decrease in numbers.

4. The detection of learning disabilities has seen phenomenal growth – an increase of 140 percent in the past decade. The increase in individuals identified as learning disabled (Algozzine and Korinek, 1985) has been accompanied by a concomitant decrease in the number of individuals labeled mildly retarded. It might also be possible that many school districts and many parents are opting to identify students as learning disabled (LD) rather than as mildly mentally retarded because the LD label is more positive and less stigmatizing. This would be encouraged because the coursework and the teaching techniques used in classrooms for students labeled LD are very similar to the coursework and techniques used in classrooms for students who are mildly retarded (Marston, 1987). Given the opportunity for a less stigmatizing label but similar types

of coursework, many parents are opting to have higher functioning students labeled LD rather than EMR. While the legality of such practices on the part of the school districts is questionable, they are seen by some as very practical and humanistic.

The lowering of the IQ cutoff for mental retardation, the addition of adaptive behavior testing, the increased diagnosis of learning disabilities, and racial discrimination issues have defined a group of mentally retarded individuals (especially mildly mentally retarded people) who are very different from those labeled EMR 15 years ago. The individuals now labeled EMR are "a more patently disabled group" (MacMillan and Borthwick, 1980, p. 157) needing more intensive individualized instruction than groups labeled mildly retarded in the past and experiencing more problems and more severe problems than their equally labeled counterparts of two decades ago.

Federal Legislation Relating to People with Mental Retardation

The Providence, Rhode Island, public schools established programs for students labeled EMR about a century ago, in 1896 (Kirk and Gallagher, 1989). Uniform provision of services to all students identified as retarded, however, was not available until the enactment of the Education of All Handicapped Children Act of 1975, the Education of All Handicapped Children Act Amendments of 1986, the Rehabilitation Act of 1973, and the Americans with Disabilities Act of 1990.

The Education of All Handicapped Children Act (EAHCA) became law in 1975 and included six major provisions:

1. "Free appropriate public education." This mandates that all children, regardless of their handicap or of the severity of that handicap, receive public, free, and appropriate education.

2. Nondiscriminatory assessment. This mandates that testing be done in an individual's native mode of communication or native tongue and that testing procedures take into account an individual's perceived area of disability. For example, a student who is blind would not be given a test that would require the student to look at objects.

3. Parental participation. The EAHCA gives parents the right to review their child's records and to approve or disapprove any placement as well as the type of educational programming.

4. Due process. Through the provisions of the EAHCA, students have a right to legal remedies in the court system if they or their guardians perceive violations of the law.

5. "Least restrictive environment." Potentially very important to librarians, this provision mandates that the environment in which disabled individuals are taught be one that provides them with the most contact with their nondisabled peers. This provision has been put into action as "mainstreaming," the process of educating disabled individuals within the regular classroom. The Eleventh Annual Report to Congress (1989) says that 86 percent of all students labeled mentally retarded spend some time each day in the regular education program. Indeed, an average of 1.3 hours per day, or 22 percent of the school day, is spent with nonhandicapped peers. The areas of mainstreaming most often involved are the so-called specials: art, gym, music, library, and nonacademic areas such as recess, homeroom, and lunch. It is not unusual to find a class in the library that consists of nonretarded students and one or two mildly retarded students. Children with more severe retardation may also be mainstreamed into special and nonacademic areas.

6. Individualized educational programming. Under the EAHCA, each disabled child is required to have an individualized education plan (IEP), which outlines goals and objectives for the school year, describes the extent of mainstreaming, and indicates the types of educational placement the student will receive. IEPs are to be written by all professionals involved with the educational experience of the student (including librarians), and they must be approved by parents prior to implementation.

The EAHCA was amended in 1986 by Public Law 99-457, resulting in the Education of All Handicapped Children Act Amendments of 1986. The amendments require that school districts provide special educational services to all children between the ages of three and five who are either handicapped or at risk of being handicapped. This includes many youngsters from low socioeconomic status (SES) environments who are at risk of being labeled retarded because they are not exposed to language, interaction, and other forms of stimulation.

The Rehabilitation Act of 1973 mandates that any agency receiving federal dollars cannot discriminate against otherwise qualified persons with handicaps. Persons with mental retardation qualify as handicapped under the Rehabilitation Act of 1973 and, therefore, must receive aid, benefits, or services that are equal to those provided to people without handicaps (Thomas, 1985).

Although the Rehabilitation Act of 1973 does not entitle a person to a job or service, it mandates public agencies to take steps to ensure that people with handicaps have available to them the variety of programs and services available to nonhandicapped people in the area served by the agency. Rothstein (1990) points out that this can include any program – for example, library or vocational education – in which people without handicaps participate. A recent case before the Office of Civil Rights (OCR), the body responsible for overseeing the enforcement of the Rehabilitation Act of 1973, involved a group of students who were labeled EMR and TMR (*Green Bay Area (Wisc.) School District*, 1990) and who were being served in self-contained special education classrooms. For some reason, they had been denied library instruction and library services even though every other student in the building received library instruction and services. The OCR ruled that the students labeled EMR and TMR had been discriminated against because they had been denied the library services that had been given to all other students. As a result, the students were given access to library instruction and library services. It should be noted that the library instruction for the students labeled EMR and TMR did not have to be identical to the instruction for nonhandicapped students; it just had to be provided. Even if mentally retarded individuals are segregated, they have the right to participate in all activities and programs offered to persons without handicaps.

Unfortunately, the impact of the Rehabilitation Act of 1973 was greatly minimized because it applied only to programs receiving federal financial assistance. To rectify this and to expand the numbers affected by the provisions of the Rehabilitation Act, the Congress passed the Americans with Disabilities Act of 1990, which guarantees that persons with disabilities, including those with mental retardation, have access to all buildings, workplaces, transportation, and telephones. The act applies to all facilities and programs, regardless of whether or not they receive federal financial aid.

Legislation has attempted to ensure that the civil rights of people with mental retardation and other disabilities are protected. Legislation has also ensured that people with mental retardation and other disabilities have access to any services available to their nonhandicapped peers, including the services and programs of a library.

Characteristics of Mentally Retarded Individuals

A number of characteristics can be identified that differentiate the mentally retarded.

1. More males than females are classified as mentally retarded (Epstein, Polloway, Patton, and Foley, 1989; McLaren and Bryson, 1987). This stems in part from a higher frequency of sex-linked disorders, causing mental retardation of males. In the past, this difference has also been attributed to the differential socialization of males and females. Because males were taught to be aggressive and to stand up for themselves, while girls were taught to be dainty and demure, the aggressive mobile boys were more likely to be noticed than the quiet girls.

2. Mentally retarded individuals, as children, often suffer from lack of stimulation. Research has shown that the lack of toys and books in a child's environment can contribute to mental retardation problems (Capron and Duyme, 1989) by limiting the opportunities of a developing child to explore, to develop cause-and-effect relationships, and to experience a variety of different materials (Elardo, Bradley, and Caldwell, 1975.

3. Mentally retarded individuals, as children, often suffer from a lack of exposure to complex communication. In some homes, conversation may encompass few abstract and multisyllable words and may be based on an informal language code that is very dissimilar to the language used in schools and on tests of intelligence. Limited exposure to formal language has been correlated with lower scores on tests of intelligence and with poor performance in school (Ramey and Macphee, 1985; Sattler, 1982).

4. Mentally retarded individuals often suffer the consequences of a lack of prenatal care. A positive correlation has been found between the amount of prenatal care received and the incidence of mild mental retardation (Broman, Nichols, Shaughnessy, and Kennedy, 1987), a result of increased rates of premature birth, and labor complications. Underweight and undernourished babies, born without benefit of adequate prenatal care, are at greater risk for delays in development. If undernourishment continues throughout childhood, the child is at risk for significantly slowed growth of the brain and brain cells.

5. Mentally retarded individuals develop at a slow rate. Persons who are mentally retarded develop at a slower rate than their nonretarded peers in the areas of language, academics, social skills, and self-help skills. The more severe the retardation disorder, the more slowly the retarded individual will develop. It is important to

note that mentally retarded people *do* develop and mature but that they do so more slowly than their nonretarded peers.

6.   Speech and language development is slow. Speech and language problems are listed as the greatest secondary handicaps among school age students identified as mentally retarded (Epstein, Polloway, Patton, and Foley, 1989). The speech and language problems of mildly retarded individuals, including difficulty with articulation and mild language problems, are usually resolved by adulthood. The problems of severely retarded individuals are more serious in nature and continue throughout the life span.

7.   Academic achievement is low. Persons who are mildly mentally retarded typically display low academic achievement, which is often the difficulty that triggers concern on the part of parents and educators and testing and identification of a person as mildly mentally retarded. Often, children are not identified as EMR until they get to school. Polloway and Smith (1986) report that the average age at identification is 5.5 years.

8.   Reading skills are low. Reading appears to be the most problematic academic area for mentally retarded individuals. Reading levels of adults with mild mental retardation vary greatly, ranging from a primer level to a sixth-grade level (Howard and Orlansky, 1988). Westling (1986) further notes that although mildly retarded adults may be able to read orally at the third- or fourth-grade level, they may have great difficulty understanding what they have read. In spite of their low reading levels, 5.8 percent of all individuals who are mentally retarded enroll at postsecondary institutions following completion of high school. The majority enroll at trade or technical schools, while a small percentage take coursework at two-year and four-year colleges and universities (11th Annual Report to Congress, 1989). Even with specific vocational training, people who are mentally retarded may be hampered by poor reading skills as they search for employment. They may not know how to go about getting a job, they may be unable to read advertisements for help, or they may not know what to do to maintain a job.

9.   Functional mental skills are often adequate. Functional mental skills – the skills that involve academics and cognitive processes – are manifested in typical everyday skills such as reading recipes, phone books, and help-wanted ads or using numerical concepts to count

change and to tell time. In a survey of parents of mildly mentally retarded individuals conducted by the Office of Special Education Programs (OSEP), 42 percent reported that their sons and daughters could perform functional mental skills either very well or pretty well (11th Annual Report to Congress, 1989). It is important to note that this survey included parents of individuals with a wide range of retardation–from mild to profound. Despite this range, 26.5 percent of the persons were reported to have functional mental skills scores of 13-15 years, while another 29.4 percent had functional mental scores of 9-12 years. These functional mental skills scores do not indicate that the persons are childlike (Patton, Beirne-Smith, and Payne, 1990) but rather that in some aspects of their lives, most notably academically oriented areas, these individuals are not as skilled as most adults, behaving instead at the indicated age level.

10. Social/emotional behavior is below average. Because mentally retarded individuals develop more slowly socially than their nonretarded peers, social problems occur and become more apparent as mentally retarded people age. For example, mildly mentally retarded children may be generally accepted by and even popular with classmates in elementary school, but they are more likely to be rejected and to become less popular as they age (Polloway, Epstein, Patton, Cullinan, and Luebke, 1986). Researchers (Polloway, Epstein, and Cullinan, 1985) also report lower self-esteem among these students. This may be because they are increasingly segregated from the mainstream as they age and as academic discrepancies become more apparent. Mildly mentally retarded individuals also exhibit more so-called behavior problems than the norm. Greater rates of disruptive behavior, attention problems, overactivity, and distractibility have been reported among the population of mildly mentally retarded individuals (Polloway and Smith, 1985). This may be explained in part by the reasons just stated and also by a complex of other possibilities: Mildly retarded individuals have difficulty distinguishing between appropriate and inappropriate behavior, are frustrated by repeated failures, or are trying to gain the attention or the approval of others by acting out.

11. Self-care is adequate. Although most mildly retarded individuals are somewhat slower in developing self-care skills, by adolescence or adulthood they are capable of performing self-care skills. In the same OSEP survey reported earlier, 67.4 percent of the parents reported that their offspring could perform self-care skills very well,

while 20.6 percent reported that their offspring could perform self-care skills pretty well (11th Annual Report to Congress, 1989).

Universal Needs of Mentally Retarded Individuals

Persons who are mentally retarded have a wide range of needs, the most common being needs for special education programming, needs for vocational education and training, needs for reader or technological services, and needs to overcome stereotypical treatment.

Special Education. Retarded individuals require varying degrees of special education programming. Because they acquire academic skills more slowly, mildly retarded individuals require slower-paced instruction, many opportunities for drill and practice, much repetition, and specialized instruction in reading and reading comprehension.

Methods for providing special education are varied, as are the modes. Most typical are self-contained, segregated classes (for individuals who learn too slowly to be accommodated in a class with nonretarded peers) and partially segregated classes (for individuals who require some special help but whose rate of learning does not require totally segregated educational programming). Another mode, called *regular education initiative*, provides all special education within an integrated classroom. Retarded and nonretarded peers are taught by the same instructor, using individualized instructional methodologies. The regular education initiative mode is very controversial but is gaining ground in many areas of the country (Davis, 1989).

Vocational Education. Without vocational training, many individuals who are mentally retarded do not obtain employment. The Eleventh Annual Report to Congress (1989) reported that 19.8 percent of adults with mental retardation who had been out of school for at least one year were employed full-time, and 11.6 percent were employed part-time. Approximately 70 percent were unemployed. In addition, even if employed, mentally retarded individuals are often the first to be laid off in times of economic recession or uncertainty.

Difficulties with job placement and employment may be exacerbated by the fact that many students with mental retardation exit school without receiving a diploma or certificate of completion. The 11th Annual Report stated that 39 percent of mentally retarded students received neither a diploma nor some type of certification of attendance, competency, or completion. They had, in essence, dropped out of school. Of this group, 26.3 percent dropped out because they had poor grades and weren't doing well in school, and 24.9 percent dropped out because they did not like school.

Poor job skills, brought about by lack of vocational training and exacerbated by lack of a diploma, have caused much hardship in the lives of people who are mentally retarded. Many adults who are mentally retarded live marginally, often in poor neighborhoods, in marginal housing, "on the edge of poverty" (Kaufman, 1988, p. 209), and with no decent health care. The OSEP survey cited earlier (11th Annual Report to Congress, 1989) stated that while 88 percent of the offspring could take care of themselves adequately, only 52.1 percent were expected to live independently. This discrepancy may be traced in part to reluctance on the part of many parents to permit their offspring to live in such marginal environments.

Reader and Technological Services. Reader and technological services may be needed by individuals who are mentally retarded. Mentally retarded persons may require someone to read materials to them or to provide help with technological services that involve the use of specialized equipment to provide access to printed material in alternative formats. Such equipment includes, but is not limited to, recorded books, computers that convert print into digitized speech, and computers that convert speech into text. The 11th Annual Report to Congress (1989) reported that, surprisingly, of the 49,469 students with mental retardation who exited school during the 1986-1987 school year, only 895 (1.8 percent) were reported to need reader services after graduation. Only 824 students (1.6 percent) were reported to need technological support services after graduation. Although these figures are surprising when one considers the difficulty individuals with mental retardation have with reading, they may also reflect ignorance on the part of secondary special educators as to what reader and technological services entail and how they may benefit persons who are retarded, or they may be explained by the lack of further contact mentally retarded persons have with reading and technological equipment.

Combating Stereotypical Treatment. Individuals who are mentally retarded may be viewed as sinister or evil, childlike, nonsexual, sex starved, burdensome, pitiable, or incapable of fully participating in daily life (Biklen and Bogdan, 1978; Bogdan and Biklen, 1977). While all of these stereotypes are incorrect, they are based on labels and preconceived notions about what retardation means (Bogdan and Taylor, 1976). They are reinforced and perpetuated by the various media – film, television, and print.

Reflect for a moment on Lennie in John Steinbeck's *Of Mice and Men*, on Dopey in Walt Disney's *Snow White and the Seven Dwarfs*, or on Charlie in Daniel Keys's *Flowers for Algernon*. All of these individuals were retarded and were portrayed as common stereotypes. When mental retardation is linked by the media to inappropriate stereotypical images, the general public begins to believe the stereotypes (Bogdan and Knolls, 1988). As a result, people with mental retardation have been and continue to be treated inappropriately, experiencing abuse, neglect, involuntary sterilization,

isolation in warehouselike institutions for decades, and denial of the right to vote, to receive education, to obtain employment, and to live independently. They have not been afforded the opportunities to do things that nonretarded people take for granted.

It is important to remember that the stereotypes are just that – *stereotypes*. Mentally retarded individuals are not to be seen as stupid (Kaufman, 1988). They merely develop at a slower rate than their nonretarded peers. They deserve to be treated as human beings with distinct personalities. As Westling (1986) notes: "Mentally retarded people do not want to be mentally retarded or considered mentally retarded. They want to be normal; they want to work; and they want to have friends. In other words, they want to be like others" (19-20).

Provision of Library Services to People Who Are Mentally Retarded

Perhaps more than any other group, librarians must develop an attitude that allows them to provide library services proactively to mentally retarded individuals. Too often, a mentally retarded patron is met with a disapproving library professional who questions the patron's ability to understand and comply with the responsibilities of library card holders. Although denial of library cards to mentally retarded individuals is illegal, it happens often, as do other forms of discrimination that result in the denial of access to library services. It is critical that librarians recognize the abilities of mentally retarded patrons and compensate in part, as described below, for their disabilities.

Collection Development. Reading is the most problematic academic area for mentally retarded individuals (with reading levels ranging from primer to sixth grade). Special attention must be paid to collection development. Certain kinds of materials are especially useful:

1. Multimedia materials. Sound/captioned filmstrips are useful and are better than silent captioned filmstrips in which the captions will be difficult for mentally retarded individuals to read. Also helpful are book-record and book-cassette kits, which allow someone with a lower reading level to comprehend at a higher reading level and which help raise the individual's reading level by increasing sight vocabulary through the hearing of the written words.

2. High interest/low vocabulary materials. Although some mentally retarded persons may read at a sixth-grade level, their interests will often be at a much higher chronological grade/age level. High interest/low vocabulary materials present complex subjects that

might interest adults (for example, books about parenting) but that are written at the reading level, for example, of a sixth grader. It is important to include educational materials, but it is just as important to include fiction, self-help, and other kinds of materials in the hi/low format. The American Library Association publishes lists of appropriate hi/low materials, and the literature of librarianship often includes criteria for selecting such materials. As with any material, criteria to ensure quality are important.

3. Highly visual print materials. Magazines and books with pictures and larger print are helpful. It is important that neither the pictures nor the print be at a baby's or young child's level (unless the book is for a baby or a young child).

4. Supplementary materials to reinforce or introduce academic subjects. Often, materials that present academic subjects at a lower or less complex reading level can allow a mentally retarded individual to more easily master concepts presented in a formal classroom situation.

5. Realia. Toys, games, puzzles, pictures, posters, and other types of realia can help a mentally retarded youngster develop more quickly. They can also help an otherwise unstimulated child from testing at a retardation level. A circulating collection of realia can help many families of mentally retarded children provide a variety of these types of expensive materials.

6. Audiovisual materials. Audiovisual materials such as films and videos (both educational and recreational) are of special interest to mentally retarded patrons. Their multimedia nature and the fact that their enjoyment does not require reading can help to reinforce the development of appropriate speech and language patterns.

Library Orientation and Bibliographic Instruction. Speech and language problems have been identified as the greatest secondary handicap of mentally retarded individuals. Individuals with speech and language problems may have difficulty following the typical fast pace of a library tour or a bibliographic instruction unit. Slower-paced and shorter tours; bibliographic instruction that emphasizes repetition, a multisensory approach to learning, noncompetitive outcomes assessment, and demonstration rather than description; and extra time for synthesis are preferable. Mentally retarded patrons may also need help applying for library cards or using the card catalog. Some librarians provide specially designed library instruction for classes of mentally retarded individuals from residential facilities and sheltered workshops.

Discipline. Because mentally retarded individuals may not have the same highly developed social skills as their nonretarded peers, they may require more attention from authority figures. For example, moderately retarded adults in the library may, at times, require one-on-one interaction with the librarian or other service provider. With this interaction, they can benefit from library services without being disruptive. It is important to acknowledge inappropriate behavior with positive discipline and to provide suitable alternative study locations, if necessary. For example, library carrels can be very helpful for mentally retarded patrons who are easily distracted, and viewing booths can be provided if the materials being used require audible or other responses that might disturb patrons.

Information and Referral. Librarians can be especially helpful to retarded (as well as to nonretarded) patrons through the provision of information and referral services to other resources. Some librarians maintain up-to-date files of local, state, and national organizations and agencies; some maintain general information resource collections about retardation; some proactively sponsor programs about retardation. All of these services fill a great need in every community to disseminate information about retardation, sources of advocacy, housing, educational alternatives and rights, vocational education, and job placement.

Programming. Typical library programs that involve films, dramatics, arts and crafts, hobbies, holidays, puppetry, and storytelling are particularly appealing to mentally retarded individuals. Literacy and reading readiness programs are useful and may be well attended.

Reader's Advisor. It is important to encourage mentally retarded individuals to select their own reading materials. Librarians may want to help by suggesting more appropriate resources on topics that a mentally retarded patron has selected or by extending the library's normal loan period to allow extra time for reading or viewing.

Organizations That Can Provide Information and Help

American Association of Mental Retardation
1719 Kalorama Road, NW
Washington, DC 20009

With a membership of physicians, educators, social workers, psychologists, psychiatrists, and others interested in the welfare of mentally retarded individuals, the association studies the causes, treatment, and prevention of mental retardation. It publishes *Mental Retardation* and the *American Journal on Mental Retardation*.

Association for Children with Downs Syndrome
2616 Martin Avenue
Bellmore, NY 11710

The association acts as a resource and information center about Downs syndrome.

Association for Children with Retarded Mental Development
162 Fifth Avenue, 11th floor
New York, NY 10010

This group of professionals, parents, and others interested in mentally retarded and developmentally disabled children and adults offers programs and workshops and acts as an advocate for mentally retarded individuals.

Association for Persons with Severe Handicaps
7010 Roosevelt Way, NE
Seattle, WA 98115

Comprised of professionals, parents, and persons with severe handicaps, the association acts as an advocate on behalf of persons with severe handicaps. It also serves as a clearinghouse of materials for individuals with severe handicaps and publishes the *Journal of the Association for Persons with Severe Handicaps*.

Association for Retarded Citizens
PO Box 6109
Arlington, TX 76005

Active promotion of services, research, public understanding, and legislation focused on the problems of mentally retarded individuals is the focus of the association.

Council for Exceptional Children
Division on Mental Retardation
2372 E. Broadmoor
Springfield, MO 65804

The division's goal is to advance the education and general welfare of mentally retarded individuals. It publishes *Education and Training in Mental Retardation*.

Federation for Children with Special Needs
95 Berkeley Street
Boston, MA 02116

This coalition of parents' organizations provides information on special education laws and resources as well as on procedures to obtain related services.

Mental Retardation Association of America
211 East 300 South, Suite 212
Salt Lake City, UT 84111

As an independent volunteer organization, the association promotes research, serves as an advocate, and sponsors public educational research.

National Association of Developmental Disabilities Councils
1234 Massachusetts Avenue, NW
Suite 103
Washington, DC 20005

The association acts as an information clearinghouse and works to educate, inform, and foster cooperation among federal, state, and volunteer organizations. It publishes *Forum*.

References

Algozzine, B., and L. Korinek. 1985. "Where Is Special Education for Students with High Prevalence Handicaps Going?" *Exceptional Children* 51: 388-94.

Bijou, S. 1966. "A Functional Analysis of Retarded Development." In *International Review of Research in Mental Retardation*, edited by N.R. Ellis, vol.1, 1-19. New York: Academic Press.

Biklen, D., and R. Bogdan. 1977. "Media Portrayals of Disabled People: A Study in Stereotypes." *Interracial Books for Children Bulletin* 8, nos. 6 and 7: 4-9.

Bogdan, R., and D. Biklen. 1977. "Handicapism." *Social Policy*, March/April, 14-19.

Bogdan, R., and J. Knoll. 1988. "The Sociology of Disability." In *Exceptional Children and Youth*. 3d ed. edited by E. L. Meyen and T. M. Skrtic. Denver: Love Publishing.

Bogdan, R., and S. Taylor. 1976. "The Judged, Not the Judges – An Insider's View of Mental Retardation." *American Psychologist* 31: 47-52.

Braveman, P., G. Oliva, M. G. Miller, R. Reiter, and S. Egerter. 1989. "Adverse Outcomes and Lack of Health Insurance among Newborns in an Eight County Area of California, 1982-1986." *New England Journal of Medicine* 321: 508-13.

Broman, S., P. L. Nichols, P. Shaughnessy, and W. Kennedy. 1987. *Retardation in Young Children*. Hillsdale, N.J.: Erlbaum.

Capron, C., and M. Duyme. 1989. "Assessment of Effects of Socio-economic Status on IQ in a Full Cross-Fostering Study." *Nature* 340: 552-54.

Davis, W. 1989. "The Regular Education Initiative: Its Promises and Problems." *Exceptional Children* 55: 440-46.

Dever, R. B. 1990. "Defining Mental Retardation from an Instructional Perspective." *Mental Retardation* 28: 147-54.

Elardo, R., R. Bradley, and B. Caldwell. 1975. "The Relation of Infants' Home Environments to Mental Test Performance from Six to Thirty-Six Months: A Longitudinal Analysis." *Child Development* 46: 71-76.

Epstein, M. H., E. A. Polloway, J. R. Patton, and R. Foley. 1989. "Mild Retardation: Student Characteristics and Services." *Education and Training in Mental Retardation* 24: 7-17.

Frankenberger, W., and J. Harper. 1988. "States' Definitions and Procedures for Identifying Children with Mental Retardation: Comparison of 1981-1982 and 1985-1986 Guidelines." *Mental Retardation* 26: 133-36.

Green Bay Area (Wisc.) School District. 16 EHLR 670 (OCR 1990).

Grossman, H. J. 1983. *Classification in Mental Retardation.* Washington, D.C.: American Association of Mental Deficiency.

Hawkins, G. D., and D. H. Cooper. 1990. "Adaptive Behavior Measures in Mental Retardation Research: Subject Description in AJMD/AJMR Articles (1979-1987)." *American Journal of Mental Retardation* 94: 654-60.

Heber, R. 1961. "A Manual on Terminology and Classification in Mental Retardation." Rev. ed. Monograph Supplement to *American Journal of Mental Deficiency*.

Heward, W. L., and M. D. Orlansky. 1988. *Exceptional Children.* Columbus, Ohio: Merrill.

Kaufman, S. Z. 1988. *Retarded ISN'T Stupid, Mom!* Baltimore: Brookes.

Kirk, S. A., and J. J. Gallagher. 1989. *Educating Exceptional Children.* 6th ed. Boston: Houghton-Mifflin.

Larry P. v. Riles. 495 F. Supp. 926 (N.D. Cal. 1979). Afff'd (9th Cir. no. 80-427, 23 Jan. 1984).

MacMillan, D. L., and S. Borthwick. 1980. "The New Educable Mentally Retarded Population: Can They Be Mainstreamed?" *Mental Retardation* 18: 155-58.

Marston, D. 1987. "Does Categorical Teacher Certification Benefit the Mildly Handicapped Child?" *Exceptional Children* 53: 423-31.

McLaren, J., and S. E. Bryson. 1987. "Review of Recent Epidemiological Studies of Mental Retardation: Prevalence, Associated Disorders, and Etiology. *American Journal of Mental Retardation* 92: 243-54.

Mercer, J. 1973. *Labelling the Mentally Retarded*. Berkeley: University of California Press.

Nihira, K., R. Foster, M. Shellhaas, and H. Leland. 1974. *AAMD Adaptive Behavior Scale*. Rev. ed. Washington, D.C.: American Association on Mental Deficiency.

Office of Special Education and Rehabilitative Services. U.S. Department of Education. 1989. *Eleventh Annual Report to Congress on the implementation of the Education of the Handicapped Act*. Washington, D.C.: Government Printing Office.

Patton, J. R., M. Beirne-Smith, and J. S. Payne. 1990. *Mental Retardation*. Columbus, Ohio: Merrill.

Polloway, E. A., M. H. Epstein, and D. Cullinan. 1985. "Prevalence of Behavior Problems among Educable Mentally Retarded Students." *Education and Training in Mental Retardation* 20: 3-13.

Polloway, E. A., M. H. Epstein, J. R. Patton, D. Cullinan, and J. Luebke. 1986. "Demographic, Social, and Behavioral Characteristics of Students with Educable Mental Retardation." *Education and Training in Mental Retardation* 21: 27-34.

Polloway, E. A., and J. D. Smith. 1987. "Current Status of the Mild Mental Retardation Construct: Identification, Placement, and Problems." In *The Handbook of Special Education: Research and Practice*, edited by M. C. Wang, M. C. Reynolds, and H. J. Wahlberg, 1-22. Oxford, England: Pergamon Press.

President's Committee on Mental Retardation. 1970. *The Six Hour Retarded Child*. Washington, D.C.: U.S. Government Printing Office.

Ramey, C. T., and D. MacPhee. 1985. "Developmental Retardation among the Poor: A Systems Theory Perspective on Risk and Prevention." In *Risk and Psychosocial Development*, edited by D. C. Farran and J. D. McKinney, 61-81. New York: Academic Press.

Reschley, D. J. 1988. "Larry P.! Larry P.! Why the California Sky Fell on IQ Testing." *Journal of School Psychology* 26:199-205.

Rothstein, L. E. 1990. *Special Education Law*. White Plains, N.Y.: Longman.

Salvia, J., and J. E. Ysseldyke. 1988. *Assessment in Special and Remedial Education*. 4th ed. Boston: Houghton-Mifflin.

Sattler, J. M. 1982. *Assessment of Children's Intelligence and Special Abilities*. Boston: Allyn and Bacon.

Sparrow, S. S., D. A. Balla, and D. V. Cicchetti. 1984. *Vineland Adaptive Behavior Scales*. Circle Pines, Minn.: American Guidance Service.

Thomas, S. 1985. *Legal Issues in Special Education*. Topeka, Kans.: NOLPE.

Thorndike, R. L., E. Hagen, and J. Sattler. 1986. *Stanford Binet Intelligence Scale*. 4th ed. Chicago: Riverside Publishing.

Wechsler, D. 1981. *Manual for Wechsler Adult Intelligence Scale*. Revised. New York: Psychological Corporation.

_____. 1974. *Wechsler Intelligence Scale for Children: Manual*. Rev. ed. New York: Psychological Corporation.

_____. 1967. *Wechsler Preschool and Primary Scale of Intelligence: Manual*. New York: Psychological Corporation.

Westling, D. 1986. *Introduction to Mental Retardation*. Englewood Cliffs, N.J.: Prentice-Hall.

Library Services to Print-Handicapped Individuals

BETH PERRY

Chief of the Regional Library for the Blind and Physically Handicapped and
User Services
Rhode Island Department of State Library Services

Definitions

Many disabilities can limit an individual's ability to read standard print. The
one that most often comes to mind is blindness, or severe visual impairment.
The legal definition of blindness, or legal blindness, is having central vision
acuity of 20/200 or less in the better eye with best correction. If acuity is
greater than 20/200, individuals are still considered legally blind if the widest
diameter of their visual field does not subtend to an angle greater than 20
degrees (Kirchner, 1988, p. 5-6). Severe visual impairment is defined as the
inability to read ordinary newspaper print even with the aid of corrective
lenses, or, if the individual is under six years of age, severe visual impairment
is defined as being blind in both eyes or having no useful vision in either eye
(Kirchner, 1988, p. 4-5).

The term *blindness* is used to include conditions such as cataracts,
where the normally transparent lens of the eye becomes cloudy or opaque;
glaucoma, where pressure of the fluid inside the eye is too high; low vision, a
persistent, irreversible deficit that interferes with daily living even with the
best optical correction provided by regular lenses; macular degeneration, or

37

deterioration of the retina; retinitis pigmentosa, a hereditary degeneration of the retina; and retinopathy of prematurity, blindness thought to be caused primarily by oxygen given to incubated premature babies (Velleman, 1990; Seligman, 1990; Johnson, 1989).

Blindness is not the only disability that can limit an individual's ability to read standard printed material. Other disabilities, including learning disabilities and physical disabilities, can also be limiting. For purposes of this chapter, visual and physical disabilities that limit a person's ability to read standard printed material are defined broadly in the context used by the National Library Service for the Blind and Physically Handicapped (NLS), which provides recorded and braille materials, free of charge, to eligible United States citizens. Within the eligibility requirements for service are the following definitions of people who qualify as unable to read standard printed material, or for purposes of this chapter, as print-handicapped:

1.   Blind persons whose visual acuity, as determined by *competent authority*, is 20/200 or less in the better eye with correcting lenses or whose widest diameter of visual field subtends an angular distance no greater than 20 degrees.

2.   Other physically handicapped persons are described as follows:

     a.   Persons whose visual disability, with correction and regardless of optical measurement, is certified by *competent authority* as preventing the reading of standard printed material.
     b.   Persons certified by *competent authority* as unable to read or unable to use standard printed material as a result of physical limitations.
     c.   Persons certified by *competent authority* as having a reading disability resulting from organic dysfunction and being of sufficient severity to prevent their reading printed material in a normal manner.

Demographics

Using the NLS definition allows a broad range of services to be provided for a great number of people. Specifically, in 1984 the National Center for Health Statistics reported that as much as 20 percent of the entire United States population had some form of disability. Of the 1979 United States civilian and noninstitutionalized population, it was estimated that approximately 18.4 million people were orthopedically impaired, 8.2 million were visually impaired, 1.6 million were impaired by missing extremities or parts of extremities, and 2.1 were million paralyzed (*Digest of Data on*

Persons with Disabilities, 1984). Of this group, it is estimated that "over three million Americans aged six or older ... are either unable to read or use regular print or have difficulty in doing so" (*A Survey to Determine the Extent of the Eligible User Population*, 1979, p. viii), and that the "incidence of persons with new print limitations is about 100,000 persons annually" (p. 10).

What these statistics indicate, more than anything, is that every librarian will encounter patrons who are print-handicapped.

Legislation

The legislation mandating service to print-handicapped individuals can be divided into several major categories.

Accessibility. The Architectural Barriers Act of 1968 (PL 90-480) mandated the elimination of architectural barriers for all handicapped persons. Later, section 502 of the Rehabilitation Act of 1973 (PL 93-112) established the Architectural and Transportation Barriers Compliance Board to ensure compliance with PL 90-480 and, in part to provide technical assistance and establish architectural accessibility standards.

Affirmative Action and Civil Rights. Section 503 of the Rehabilitation Act of 1973 (PL 93-112) prohibits discrimination of qualified handicapped individuals by federal contractors. Section 504 of the same act prohibits discrimination of handicapped individuals by any program receiving federal financial assistance. Section 501 established the Interagency Committee on Handicapped Employees to implement affirmative action programs.

Library Services. The Pratt-Smoot Act of 1931 (PL 71-787) authorized the Library of Congress to purchase books in braille to be lent to blind adults. Through amendments to the Pratt-Smoot Act and through PL 89-522, the Library of Congress services have been expanded to include the purchase and distribution of materials in braille and in all recorded formats to be lent to all qualified individuals, both children and adults. Later, the Library Services and Construction Act (PL 89-511) and its amendments (1970, 1984) provided financial assistance for state, local, and regional libraries, which would serve as distribution centers for the materials lent through the National Library Service for the Blind and Physically Handicapped of the Library of Congress.

Postage Services. The Postal Reorganization Act of 1970 (PL 93-112) provides free mailing of matter for blind and physically handicapped persons.

Special Education. The Federal Assistance to State Operated Schools for the Handicapped Act (PL 89-313) provides financial assistance for the construction and operation of elementary and secondary special educational facilities, and the Education for All Handicapped Children Act (PL 94-142) guarantees free appropriate public education, related services, and individualized instructional programs for all handicapped children.

Technology. The Educational Broadcasting Facilities and Telecommunications Demonstration Act of 1976 (PL 94-309) authorized grants to public broadcasting facilities to cover 75 percent of the costs of special radio receivers that can be tuned to subcarrier channels of FM radio stations. These stations typically are used to provide radio reading services for blind individuals who otherwise would not be able to benefit from newspapers, local retail advertising, and other written communications generally available to the sighted community. More recently, the Technology-Related Assistance for Individuals with Disabilities Act of 1988 (PL 100-407) has created competitive state grant programs to support financially the development of assistive technology devices and services for disabled people.

The most recent legislation enacted is the American Disabilities Act of 1990, which substantially broadens the scope of previous legislation and prohibits discrimination on a wider range of subjects, including private employment, public accommodation, state and local government services, transportation, and telecommunication.

Needs of Print-Handicapped Individuals

"Of all the roadblocks in the path of the blind today, one rises up more formidably and threateningly than all others. It is the invisible barrier of ingrained social attitudes toward blindness and the blind – attitudes based on suspicion and superstition, on ignorances and error, which continue to hold sway in men's minds and to keep the blind in bondage" (Jernigan, 1990, p. 344). A most pressing concern of print-handicapped individuals is, as Jernigan indicates, the ignorance of nondisabled people. It, more than anything else, is responsible for the isolation that many disabled individuals feel, and it gives rise to many of the unmet needs with which disabled individuals must constantly deal. Listed below are some of the needs specific to print-handicapped individuals, along with suggestions of ways librarians can help.

Need for Information about Print Handicaps. Through careful collection development, librarians can select balanced and unbiased materials that inform on both technical and nontechnical levels. Information is needed particularly about the causes of print handicaps and their medical and nonmedical remediation. The National Library Service for the Blind and Physically Handicapped publishes "Reference Circulars," which provide bibliographies related to collection development. *Building a Library Collection on Blindness and Physical Handicaps: Basic Materials and Resources* (1985) is particularly useful. This resource is updated quarterly by

"Added Entries," a selected list of NLS new acquisitions on handicapping conditions. Information about both can be obtained from the reference section of the NLS. (The address is in the list of agencies at the end of the chapter.)

Need for Information and Referral Services. A particular need exists for information about low-vision clinics and organizations to which ophthalmologists sometimes fail to refer patients (Seligman, 1990). Many librarians also maintain a register of local readers and transcribers who will transfer printed information onto tape or braille and who will provide reading assistance on demand.

Need for Bibliotherapeutic Materials. The reading of fiction and nonfiction in which a character is disabled can profoundly shape perceptions about disabled people. Baskin and Harris (1984) cite many benefits of bibliotherapeutic materials in contrast to or in addition to expensive group intervention strategies. Benefits include reduced costs because print and nonprint media can be borrowed through interlibrary loan; less training time because certified teachers and librarians are already educated to use literature for specific purposes; better matches between the disability and the specific materials that describe it; adaptability because books are limitlessly flexible; less labor-intensive intervention and better scheduling compatibility because books are read individually; better individualization of the intervention because so many different books are available; and longer duration because books are a lifelong habit whereas workshops and classes occur infrequently or sporadically. Also important are the wonderful opportunities that books provide individuals to identify with character models. Many lists of recommended materials that portray disabled individuals can be found in the library literature. A well-known example is Baskin and Harris's *More Notes from a Different Drummer* (1984) and their earlier *Notes from a Different Drummer* (1977).

Need for Assistive Devices. Assistive devices can help print-handicapped patrons read and librarians should either try to make them available or provide information about these devices. Among the more well known devices are:

1. Optical character recognition and synthetic speech devices. Machines that convert text into speech, large print, or tactile formats are potentially very helpful. One such device is the Kurzweil Personal Reader, a portable optical scanner that reads most typewritten material and turns it into DECtalk synthetic speech. When interfaced with other computer devices, it creates a talking terminal that is compatible with word processing, communications, and braille conversion software packages, although this may not be the best use of these programs. Sold by Kurzweil Computer

41

Products, Xerox Company,[1] the Kurzweil Personal Reader combines artificial intelligence and intelligent character recognition as it reads pages of print placed face down on a glass surface or scanned by a handheld scanner. The machine comes in portable and desktop sizes.

Telesensory Systems[2] produces similar assistive devices: OsCar is a product that performs optical character recognition (OCR) to input materials into computer files or convert text into speech, braille, or print by using an IBM-AT or compatible computer, a Navigator Versabraille II+, or a VersaPoint braille printer. Other systems such as Vert Plus, Personal Vert, Lap Vert, and Soft Vert (from Telesensory Systems, Inc.) allow blind individuals to convert computer output into speech, and some (i.e., VISTA from Telesensory) allow magnified screen output. Because these types of assistive devices allow patrons to use materials already available in the library, they have the potential of being especially useful, although some of the literature indicates that the amount of training necessary to use them effectively can be an obstacle.

2. Descriptive video service (DVS). A new technology developed by WGBH-TV, Boston, is being utilized by approximately 32 public television stations. Descriptive video is used in conjunction with regular television programming. During periods of silence on the program, a narrator describes the action, settings, scene changes, and body language that are taking place. To receive DVS, the viewer must have either a stereo TV or a stereo VCR that includes the Separate Audio Program (SAP) channel. For more information about DVS, people can contact WGBH.[3]

3. Closed-circuit television systems. By means of a camera attached to a high-resolution monitor, individuals who are visually impaired can transfer regular print into large print (up to 60 times the size of the original), with either a positive display (black letters on a white background) or a negative display (white letters on a black background), and can isolate lines of print by blocking out portions of the display. Suppliers include Telesensory Systems, Inc., Optalec,[4] and HumanWare.[5]

4. Image enlarging systems. Working within a computer, image-enlarging software allows visually impaired individuals to see the images on their computer's screen enlarged 2 to 16 times the original size. These types of systems are available from Telesensory

Systems, Optalec (LP-DOS), HFK Software (QLP-Plus),[6] and major computer manufacturers.

5. Braille conversion systems. By means of a circuit board that attaches to a Perkins Brailler and then to a computer printer, blind individuals can type in braille and produce print copies of the typed material for sighted peers. One such device is called MPRINT, available from Telesensory Systems. Another, called the Duxbury braille translation program,[7] allows a computer to translate print screen images to a braille printer.

6. Dictation to print systems. Systems such as VoiceReport (from Kurzweil Applied Intelligence[8]) convert dictation into print output via computer technology. Included among the VoiceReport products are specialty packages such as VoiceRAD (for use by radiologists), VoiceEM (used for emergency medicine), and VoicePATH (used by surgical pathologists). Other specialty packages are available for use by professionals in business, law, and government.

7. Variable speed tape players. Tape recorders and players that have variable speed control and pitch restoration are available for purchase as noted in the NLS publication *Facts: Sources for Purchase of Cassette Players Compatible with Recorded Materials Produced by the National Library Service.*

8. Magnifying glasses. These low-tech options for individuals with low vision can be purchased in a variety of sizes, magnifications, portability, and light sources. Local low vision clinics can recommend appropriate uses, and simple individual magnifying glasses can be purchased at local stores.

Need for Alternative Formats of Print Materials. Print-handicapped individuals have the same library and information needs as anyone else. Only their need for alternative formats differs from non-print-handicapped individuals. Librarians can be especially helpful in several areas.

1. Provision of large-print materials. Many print-handicapped individuals are visually impaired but not blind. This means that they can read print if it is sufficiently large and sufficiently bold. The provision of large-print (typically 14 to 30 point type) books and magazines (available from publishers such as G. K. Hall, Thorndike, and Ulverscroft) can make the difference between reading and not reading. It is encouraging that mainstream publishers are beginning

to publish their books simultaneously in regular print and in large print. Photocopiers that enlarge text for individual use are also helpful in special cases.

2. Provision of braille materials. Braille is an acceptable format for some, but by no means all, print-handicapped individuals. Although braille materials are bulky (it takes many volumes of braille to equal just one volume of print) and difficult to store (they are oversized and cannot be stored in a horizontal position because the raised dots can be crushed), the format is invaluable both for reading and for taking notes. The NLS provides braille materials as part of its loan services, and many local organizations can produce braille materials on demand. If the demand warrants it, a braille typewriter in the library can also be helpful.

3. Provision of recorded materials. Recorded fiction and nonfiction resources are heavily used by print-handicapped individuals. The NLS provides leisure-reading fiction and nonfiction through its regional library system. Recording for the Blind provides textbook materials directly to registered borrowers. Local organizations that record on demand (sometimes in sound labs within the library) can also be of help, as can local collections of commercially produced recordings. Librarians often combine recorded or braille materials (supplied by the NLS) with parallel print resources (supplied from a local library collection). This allows, for example, print-handicapped parents to read along with or to their sighted children.

4. Provision of information for current awareness in alternative formats. Unless it is provided in oral format, the news and current information found in newspapers, local printed advertising, television listings, and other local or national printed resources will not help print-handicapped individuals. Radio reading services that broadcast these types of information each day are becoming a common solution. The reading services are broadcast on an FM station's subcarrier channel and are received through an FM subcarrier receiver.

Need for Readers and Segregated Reading Areas. Because many print-handicapped individuals rely on oral formats, they may also require segregated listening rooms that will allow them to listen to materials without disturbing other patrons. The use of headphones may eliminate this need, however. Also very helpful is the provision of assistants who will read card catalog (or computerized catalog) entries, find items on the shelf, facilitate browsing by reading sections of books on demand, and provide expanded reference service by reading specific sections of reference materials on demand.

Need for Elimination of Architectural Barriers. It is particularly important to eliminate architectural barriers (i.e., stools in the middle of aisles, chairs that aren't pushed into the desk, doors that are half open). It is also important not to change the floor plan of a library unless absolutely necessary, because a blind person will have to relearn any changed floor plans.

Jean Seligman (1990) has spoken of the fear most Americans have of blindness. She asks people to "try to imagine what it is like to be a little bit blind, to live with a kind of semi-vision that even the strongest glasses can't correct. To be able to read the title of the book, but not the opening paragraph. To see the tennis players, but not the ball. And to recognize the face of a friend, but not its subtle changes of expression. Some say it's like trying to see through a thin coating of Vaseline. Others report that they view the world as if through a narrow tunnel – or a pair of glasses with missing pieces" (p. 92).

The experience is frightening, but there are many ways to help. Some have been listed. Other ideas are available from the many agencies and associations that focus on print handicaps. Some of these are listed below.

Major National Advocacy/Information Agencies

American Council of the Blind, Inc.
1155 15th Street, NW, Suite 720
Washington, DC 20005

This affiliation of individuals and organizations provides information and referral services; legal assistance and representation; scholarships; leadership and legislative training; consumer advocate support; assistance for technological research; speaker referral services; consultative and advisory services to individuals, organizations, and agencies; and program development assistance. The council publishes *The Braille Forum*.

American Foundation for the Blind, Inc.
15 West Sixteenth Street
New York, NY 10011

The foundation provides direct and technical assistance services to blind and visually impaired persons and their families, professionals in specialized agencies for the blind, community agencies, organizations, schools, and corporations. It acts as a national clearinghouse for information about blindness and visual impairment, maintains the Helen Keller Archives, and initiates and stimulates research to determine the most effective methods of serving visually impaired persons. Its National Technology Center evaluates, designs, and adapts assistive devices for visually impaired individuals, and its Radio Information Service Unit gathers and disseminates information about radio reading and information services. The foundation records and manufactures talking books and publishes the *Journal of Visual Impairment and Blindness* and the *Directory of Services for Blind and Visually Impaired Persons in the U.S.*

American Printing House for the Blind
1839 Frankfort Avenue
Louisville, KY 40206

This national organization was founded to produce literature in braille, large-type and recorded formats and to manufacture educational aids for visually impaired students. Since 1879, the American Printing House has received an annual appropriation from Congress to provide textbooks and education aids for all students attending schools and special educational institutions of lower than college grade. This money is supplemented by private donations. The American Printing House manufactures special educational aids for blind and visually handicapped persons. The organization maintains an educational research and development program in the areas of educational procedures and methods and the development of education aids. Through its Instructional Materials Center, it provides a reference-catalog service for volunteer-produced textbooks in all media for visually handicapped students and provides information about other sources of materials for those interested in the education of the visually handicapped.

Division of Blind and Visually Impaired
Rehabilitation Services Administration
U.S. Department of Education.
Room 3227
Mary E. Switzer Building
330 C Street Southwest
Washington, DC 20202

The division administers the Randolph-Sheppard Act, which assures priority for blind persons in the operation of vending facilities on federal property. It also assists the states in providing vocational rehabilitation services to blind persons to enable them to become self-supporting and gainfully employed. This includes analyzing occupations to ascertain their suitability for performance without use of sight; demonstrating to employers the suitability for employment of blind persons who are properly selected and adequately prepared for work; promoting and supporting institutes and training programs; developing, in cooperation with state agencies, new training facilities for blind persons, assisting in the expansion of existing facilities; administering the grant for the Helen Keller National Center (established to provide a national center and network for the rehabilitation of deaf-blind youth and adults); and cooperating in the development of the 7C Independent Living Services program for older blind individuals.

National Association for the Visually Handicapped, Inc.
22 West 21st Street
New York, NY 10010

The association produces and distributes large-type reading materials and informational materials to schools, libraries, senior citizen centers, hospitals, and individuals on request; assists libraries and senior centers in establishing large-print libraries; acts as an information clearinghouse and referral center regarding resources available to the partially seeing; and offers counsel and guidance to partially sighted individuals and their families.

National Federation of the Blind
1800 Johnson Street
Baltimore, MD 21230

This national federation of state and local organizations representing blind persons in the United States works to improve social and economic conditions of blind persons, focusing on their complete equality and their integration into society. It evaluates present programs, assists in establishing new ones, grants scholarships to blind persons, monitors legislation affecting the blind, supports and conducts scholarly research, conducts seminars, disseminates information, and maintains a speakers' bureau. The federation publishes the *Braille Monitor*, *Future Reflections*, and *Voice of the Diabetic*.

National Library Service for the Blind and Physically Handicapped
1291 Taylor Street, NW
Washington, DC 20542

The NLS records, manufactures, and provides, free of charge, recorded and braille materials to eligible blind and physically handicapped persons. The reading materials produced are lent through a cooperating network of 56 regional and 92 subregional libraries that circulate them to eligible borrowers by postage-free mail. Network libraries also offer reference, readers' advisory, and other services. Playback equipment is lent free for use with recorded books and magazines. Music services are provided by the NLS music section, which has an extensive collection of music scores, books, and instructional materials in braille, large-print, and recorded media. Through its reference section, the NLS serves as a national information resource on various aspects of handicapping conditions and publishes many free items, including reference circulars, that deal with aspects of print handicaps and resources for print-handicapped individuals. The NLS *Talking Book Topics* and *Magazines in Special Media* provide ongoing notices of newly recorded or brailled materials.

National Society to Prevent Blindness
500 East Remington Road
Schaumburg, IL 60173

Through state affiliates, the society conducts educational programs for laypersons and professionals, conducts research, and provides services to communities (industrial and public) to help prevent blindness. Other specific services include promotion and support of local glaucoma and preschool vision screening programs, programs on industrial eye safety, collection of statistical and other data on the nature and extent of causes of visual impairment and blindness, and medical research on visual impairment. The society publishes *Insight/Wise Owl News* and *National Society to Prevent Blindness – Insight*.

RP Foundation Fighting Blindness (formerly the National Retinitis Pigmentosa Foundation, Inc.)
1401 Mt. Royal Avenue
Fourth Floor
Baltimore, MD 21217

The foundation awards grants for research on retinitis pigmentosa and other retinal degenerative diseases, maintains a retina donor national registry program for persons with retinitis pigmentosa and their blood relatives, produces and disseminates print and nonprint information, provides referral services, and coordinates self-help networks for persons with Usher's syndrome and Laurence-Moon-Biedl syndrome.

Recording for the Blind, Inc.
20 Roszel Road
Princeton, NJ 08540

This New Jersey-based group produces and lends taped educational textbooks at no charge (after initial $25 registration fee) to visually, perceptually, and physically impaired grade school, high school, and college students and professionals. Recording is done on demand in 28 studios across the country by over 5,000 trained volunteers. Recorded titles supplement but do not duplicate those of the NLS, and master tapes of completely recorded books are kept in the organization's library to fill future requests for the material. Approximately 4,000 recorded titles are added every year.

Notes

1. Kurzweil Computer Products, 185 Albany Street, Cambridge, MA 02139.

2. Telesensory Systems, Inc. PO Box 7455, Mountain View, CA 94039-7455.

3. Descriptive Video Service, WGBH, 125 Western Avenue, Boston, MA 02134.

4. Optalec USA Inc., 4 Liberty Way, Westford, MA 01886.

5. HumanWare Inc., 6140 Horseshoe Bar Road, Suite P, Loomis, CA 95650.

6. HFK Software, Old Danbury Road, Danbury, NH 03230.

7. Duxbury System Inc., 435 King Street, PO Box 1504, Littleton, MA 01640.

8. Kurzweil Applied Intelligence, Inc., 411 Waverly Oaks Road, Waltham, MA 02154.

References

Annual Report. 1989. Ushering in the Sixtieth Year of Service. National Library Service for the Blind and Physically Handicapped. Washington, D.C., Library of Congress.

Baskin, B. H., and K. Harris, eds. 1982. *The Mainstreamed Library: Issues, Ideas, Innovations*. Chicago: American Library Association.

Baskin, B., and K. Harris. 1984. *More Notes from a Different Drummer*. New York: Bowker.

Dequin, H. C. 1983. *Librarians Serving Disabled Children and Young People*. Littleton, Colo.: Libraries Unlimited.

Digest of Data on Persons with Disabilities. 1984. Prepared under contract to Congressional Research Service, Library of Congress, Mathematical Policy Research, Inc. John L. Czajka, principal investigator. Washington, D.C.: U.S. Department of Education.

Directory of Services for Blind and Visually Impaired Persons in the United States. 1988. New York: American Foundation for the Blind.

Facts: Cassette Magazines Produced by Network Libraries. December 1989. Washington, D.C., National Library Service for the Blind and Physically Handicapped, Library of Congress.

Facts: Sources for Purchase of Cassette Players Compatible with Recorded Materials Produced by the National Library Service (NLS). October 1989. Washington, D.C., National Library Service for the Blind and Physically Handicapped, Library of Congress.

Guide to Spoken-Word Recordings: Popular Literature. Reference Circular no. 87-1. February 1987. Washington, D.C., National Library Service for the Blind and Physically Handicapped, Library of Congress.

Hollmann, F. W. 1980. *United States Population Estimates by Age, Sex, Race, and Hispanic Origin: 1980 to 1988.* Current Population Reports Series P-25, no. 1045. Washington, D.C., U.S. Department of Commerce, Bureau of the Census.

Jernigan, K. 1990. "Blindness: The Myth and the Image." *Illinois Libraries* 72, no. 4 (April): 344.

Johnson, L. 1989. "Let's Teach Grade One Braille." *Journal of Visual Impairment and Blindness* 83 (December): 491.

Kirchner, C. 1985. *Data on Blindness and Visual Impairment in the U.S.: A Resource Manual on Characteristics, Education, Employment and Service Delivery.* New York: American Foundation for the Blind.

Kirchner, C. 1988. *Data on Blindness and Visual Impairment in the U.S.: A Resource Manual on Social Demographic Characteristics, Education, Employment and Income, and Service Delivery.* New York: American Foundation for the Blind.

"Library Services for Persons with Handicaps." 1990. *Illinois Libraries* 72, no. 4 (April): entire issue.

Lovejoy, E. G. 1990. *Portraits of Library Service to People with Disabilities.* Boston: G. K. Hall.

Mandelbaum, J. B. 1989. "READS [Reader Enrollment and Delivery System]: A Networked PC System." *Information Technology and Libraries* 8 (June): 196-202.

McCormick, E. 1990. "Volunteers to Produce Braille on Demand from Floppy Disks." *American Libraries* 21 (February): 99.

National Library Service for the Blind and Physically Handicapped. 1989. *Library Resources for the Blind and Physically Handicapped: A Directory* with *FY 1988 Statistics and Readership, Circulation, Budget, Staff, and Collections*. Washington, D.C.: Library of Congress.

National Library Service for the Blind and Physically Handicapped. 1989. *News* 20 (January-March).

Occupational Outlook Handbook, 1986-87. 1988. Washington, D.C.: U.S. Department of Labor, Bureau of Labor Statistics.

Prine, S. 1989. "Blind and Physically Handicapped, Library Service to." In *The ALA Yearbook of Library and Information Services*, edited by R. Parent, 77-78. Chicago: American Library Association.

Reading Materials in Large Type. Reference Circular no. 87-4. July 1987. Washington, D.C.: National Library Service for the Blind and Physically Handicapped, Library of Congress.

Reading, Writing, and Other Communication Aids for Visually and Physically Handicapped Persons. Reference Circular, no. 86-4. August 1986. Washington, D.C.: National Library Service for the Blind and Physically Handicapped, Library of Congress.

Seligman, J. 1990. "Making the Most of Sight: A Brighter Future for the Millions of Americans with 'Low Vision.'" *Newsweek* 115 (16 April): 92-93.

Siegel, J. S., and M. Davison. August 1984. *Demographic and Socioeconomic Aspects of Aging in the United States*. Current Population Reports, Series P. 23, no. 138. Washington, D.C.: U.S. Department of Commerce, Bureau of the Census.

Statistical Abstract of the United States 1989: National Data Book and Guide to Sources. 1989. Washington, D.C.: U.S. Department of Commerce, Bureau of the Census.

Statistical Abstract of the United States 1990: National Data Book and Guide to Sources. 1990. Washington, D.C.: U.S. Department of Commerce, Bureau of the Census.

A Survey to Determine the Extent of the Eligible User Population Not Currently Being Served by the National Library Service for the Blind and Physically Handicapped. 1979. New York: American Foundation for the Blind.

Taeuber, C. M. September 1983. *America in Transition: An Aging Society*. Current Population Reports Series P-23, no. 128. Washington, D.C.: U.S. Department of Commerce, Bureau of the Census.

That All May Read: Library Service for Blind and Physically Handicapped People. 1983. Washington, D.C.: National Library Service for the Blind and Physically Handicapped, Library of Congress.

U.S. Senate Special Committee on Aging in Conjunction with the American Association of Retired Persons. 1984. *Aging America: Trends and Projections*. Washington, D.C.: American Association of Retired Persons.

Velleman, R. A. 1990. *Meeting the Needs of People with Disabilities: A Guide for Librarians, Educators, and Other Service Professionals*. Phoenix: Oryx Press.

Wright, K. C., and J. F. Davie. 1989. *Library and Information Services for Handicapped Individuals*. Englewood, Colo.: Libraries Unlimited.

Library Services to Deaf or Hearing Impaired Individuals

PHYLLIS I. DALTON

Library consultant and author of *Library Service to the Deaf and Hearing Impaired*

Introduction

A deaf or hearing impaired person is one who cannot hear or who cannot hear accurately or distinctly. Deaf individuals are unable to understand speech owing to a total loss of hearing, while hearing impaired individuals (also referred to as hard of hearing) have difficulty understanding speech because of a partial loss of hearing. More than 10 percent of the entire population of the United States is deaf or hearing impaired, which translates into a group of over 23 million people, over 3 million of whom are deaf.

In this discussion, the deaf community is interpreted as including American Sign Language (ASL) users, sign language users, bilingual users (people who are fluent in both the spoken word and sign language), oralists (people whose primary communication mode is speech and lipreading), people with minimal language skills (those who have a limited knowledge of both the spoken word and sign language), people who use total communication (a combination of signing, speaking, lipreading, and writing), deafened adults (people who lost their hearing after having finished their education but before the aging process), hearing impaired elderly (people who have a hearing loss because of the aging process), hard of hearing individuals (people with a defective but functioning sense of hearing), and hearing persons with deaf or hearing impaired family members.

Federal Legislation Relating to People with a Hearing Loss

Federal, state, and local legislation specifically mandating library service to people with a hearing loss is nonexistent. While there are many reasons for this, probably the three most important factors are (1) A hearing loss is, for the most part, an invisible disability that often goes unrecognized; (2) a hearing loss tends to isolate people so that they are less visible to the general public; and (3) people who are deaf or hearing impaired traditionally have not formed cohesive groups that could ensure the enactment of legislation.

Although library service to people who are deaf or hearing impaired is not mandated, several federal laws do relate specifically to people who are deaf or hearing impaired, and other general legislation has included deaf or hearing impaired people within the disabilities cited. These laws assist in the provision of library service even though such service is not named in the provisions of the acts. The major legislation of this type can be categorized into several areas.

Housing. In 1989, the Fair Housing Amendments of 1988 (FHA) were signed into law. This marked the first major substantive law in which discrimination in housing on the basis of disability was prohibited. It also marked the first major substantive civil rights federal law in which discrimination on the basis of disability was added to other prohibited civil rights discrimination. Among the provisions of the FHA of 1988 are the setting up of accessibility standards for the design and construction of housing and the provision to allow individuals with disabilities to make reasonable modifications in a rented dwelling at their own expense if such modifications are necessary for full enjoyment of the premises. Enforcement of the FHA's provisions is provided for because the act allows judges to levy substantial fines for failure to observe its provisions.

Education. In 1857, Gallaudet College (Washington, DC) was founded. The college became a university in 1986. Gallaudet remains the only university in the United States that provides education and resources specifically, and almost exclusively, for deaf or hearing impaired people. It offers both undergraduate and graduate programs and serves as a research facility and clearinghouse specializing in the area of deafness.

In 1965, the (NTID) National Technical Institute for the Deaf (Rochester, NY) was established. Part of the Rochester Institute of Technology, the NTID is the first effort to educate large numbers of deaf students within a college campus planned primarily for hearing students. Its unique programs are not offered anywhere else in the world. It provides technical education and training to deaf students in accessible formats and conducts applied research into the social, educational, and economic needs of deaf student populations. In the summer of 1990, NTID opened its doors to international deaf students.

In 1986, the Commission on Education of the Deaf was established under the Federal Education of the Deaf Act of 1986. Mandated to study the quality of U.S. educational programs serving individuals who are deaf, the commission's report, entitled "Toward Equality: Education of the Deaf," was submitted to Congress and the President in 1988. Among the subjects it addresses are illiteracy among deaf persons; the impact of deafness on reading skills, job opportunities, and advancement in the workplace; and language acquisition of deaf or hearing impaired students during elementary and secondary education. The long-term results of this report will ensure, without a doubt, improved education for people who are deaf.

The most important legislation, historically, affecting the education of students with disabilities is the Education for All Handicapped Children's Act (1975), PL 94-142. It guarantees appropriate education to every child in the least physically restrictive environment. As a result of this act, mainstreaming has become the preferred educational method in public schools for many students who are deaf or hearing impaired. Further, the act has facilitated the development of programs in publicly supported schools for the deaf in the majority of the states.

Section 504 of the Rehabilitation Act of 1973 is equally important to deaf students because it helps ensure that they have equal access to postsecondary education, in part by mandating the provision of interpreters for students. Because of PL 94-142 and Section 504, public schools cannot deny a child with a disability an education.

Three other older acts that should be noted are the Elementary and Secondary Education Act of 1965, the Higher Education Act of 1965, and the Vocational Education Act of 1963.

The Elementary and Secondary Education Act of 1965 initially represented federal commitment to the improvement of elementary and secondary education. Full funding for state-operated and -supported schools for handicapped children was mandated under the 1967 amendments to the act. In 1981, when Congress enacted the Education Consolidation and Improvement Act, many more beneficial changes were made in the law, especially those that increased the control local education officials have over programs for educationally deprived children.

The Higher Education Act became law in 1965. It helped establish a national policy of increasing the accessibility of postsecondary education to disadvantaged students. In the process, several provisions were included that directly or indirectly benefit people who are disabled, especially the recognition that access to postsecondary educational opportunities was limited for disabled adults and should be enhanced.

The Vocational Education Act of 1963 (with amendments) has enabled youth with handicapping conditions to receive basic vocational education. Administration of federal funds under this act requires that people with disabilities receive equal access in recruitment, enrollment, and placement activities.

Employment. The principal federal statute relating to employment of people with disabilities is the Rehabilitation Act of 1973, whose provisions prohibit discrimination by employers with federal contracts or with federal funding and require employers to take action to employ people with disabilities. Employers who have federal contracts or who receive federal funding cannot refuse to accommodate or hire a qualified person who is disabled.

A second act, the Job Training Partnership Act of 1982 as amended (JPTA), has as its basic aim to train and place "economically disadvantaged" persons in the work force through joint public-private sector initiative. This has benefited deaf or hearing impaired people because the tern *economically handicapped* includes adults who are disabled and who meet certain economic need criteria.

For employers who wish to employ people with disabilities (including those with a hearing loss), there is the very helpful Job Accommodation Network (JAN) of the President's Committee on Employment of People with Disabilities. Still another program that can be helpful is the Vocational Rehabilitation On the Job Training Program. The incentive for companies to participate is that under this program payment of disabled employee's wages is shared by the government for a limited time on a negotiated schedule. The employee must be a Vocational Rehabilitation client, and the position must be permanent, must be full time, and must pay the minimum wage. A final valuable program is the Fair Labor Standards Act of 1935 (amended 1966, 1977, 1986). This act, in addition to its general provisions establishing the minimum federal requirement for hours of work and equitable wages, includes special provisions governing the employment of people who are disabled. People with a hearing loss benefit from both the general and special provisions.

Technology. The first phase of the Hearing Aid Compatibility Act of 1988 went into effect in 1989. This act requires that all corded telephones manufactured or imported for installation in the United States for public use be hearing-aid compatible (HAC) and that all cordless telephones be HAC by 1991.

In 1988, the Technology-Related Assistance for Individuals with Disabilities Act of 1988 was signed into law. Responding to findings that technology can provide important tools to help all individuals perform tasks more easily and more quickly and that assistive technology is a necessity for some individuals with disabilities, the act provides financial assistance for states to develop and implement programs of technology-related assistance for disabled individuals. The provision of communication devices for deaf or hearing impaired individuals has been greatly facilitated by this law, as well as by the 1990 passage of the Television Decoder Circuitry Act of 1989, which mandates that captioning capability be built into television sets sold in the United States beginning in 1993.

An older act of interest in this category is the Captioned Films for the Deaf Act, enacted by Congress in 1958. The act allowed the Office of Education to purchase, lease, or accept films; provide captions for them; and distribute them through state schools and other appropriate agencies. Amendments to the act in 1962 authorized the production of captioned films, the training of persons in their use, and the conduct of research to improve the quality and effectiveness of production. The act and its amendments facilitate broad utilization of the film medium. In 1967, the act's authority was broadened to include forms of instruction such as tapes and transparencies. The Education of the Handicapped Amendments of 1977 continued the program without change.

Library Services. One federal legislative act that is not mandatory but that has been invaluable to people who have a hearing loss is the Library Services and Construction Act (LSCA). Through the LSCA, disabled people have been helped in their quest for information, education, and employment. The LSCA is probably the most important source of federal funding for libraries and library services in the United States. The funds available under this act are allocated by the federal government to the states; the states then award the funds for state or local projects. Among the purposes and goals of this act is to make library service accessible to persons with disabilities who are, because of accessibility problems, unable to benefit from public library service made available to the general public. Many library projects to make facilities and resources accessible to individuals who are deaf or hearing impaired have been funded through this act.

The Americans with Disabilities Act (ADA). Passed in the summer of 1990, the Americans with Disabilities Act (PL 101-336) prohibits discrimination against people with disabilities in the areas of accessibility, employment, housing, public accommodations, travel, communications, and state and local government. It is considered the most important piece of disability-related legislation ever passed, in part because it mandates compliance of companies with 15 or more employees, regardless of their source of funding. It is estimated that without this act, 90 percent of all employers could legally discriminate against people with disabilities.

Most important for people who are deaf is that the act bans discrimination and requires access to telephone service. With the passage of this bill, people who are deaf can assume use of the telephone in the same way as hearing people. The ADA requires all telephone companies to provide dual party relay services for local and long distance calls. By 1993, deaf people can expect to use Telecommunication Devices for the Deaf (TDD) to make telephone calls at any time, based on standards for the relay system set up by the Federal Communication Commission (FCC).

Another important element of the ADA is its requirement that all public service announcements for television that are produced or funded by the federal government be closed-captioned. Further, through ADA, many of the requirements of Section 504 of the Rehabilitation Act of 1973 are extended to private businesses that do not receive federal funds and to state and local government services without respect to the source of their funding. Employers are required to provide reasonable accommodations for people with disabilities, including the provision of TDDs and qualified interpreters. Access to state and local government service is required, including a direct TDD line to 911 telephone networks.

The passage of the ADA probably marks the beginning of more change. Regulations for its implementation are being written by different organizations. (For example, the Justice Department is writing the regulations covering the public accommodation section.)

Of the 43 million disabled people the ADA affects, an estimated 24 million are hearing and speech impaired. Dr. I. King Jordan, the first deaf president of Gallaudet University, has said that the ADA will give disabled individuals the same rights and opportunities that other Americans have enjoyed for the past 200 years.

Characteristics and Recognition of People Who Are Deaf or Hearing Impaired

It is not easy to recognize people who have hearing loss even though they are a part of every community. For example, a person wearing a hearing aid may actually hear quite well when there are few background noises. A hearing aid tends to exaggerate background noise; in the presence of background noises, the same hearing impaired person may not be able to hear at all. School age children who cannot hear may be misdiagnosed as mentally retarded or as having behavioral problems. Unfortunately, the children may not know that they have a hearing loss, and the perceptions of others may influence their behavior in a "self-fulfilling prophecy." Adults may be similarly misunderstood by others. They also may not realize that they have a hearing loss.

Difficulties recognizing and correctly diagnosing deafness and hearing impairment can be alleviated through knowledge of some basic characteristics that typically indicate hearing impairment. Although each person in the deaf community is truly individual, all will exhibit difficulties communicating via traditional (oral/aural) media. To varying degrees, deaf or hearing impaired people will:

1. Use some form of sign language, lipreading, or both to communicate. Depending upon the severity of the hearing loss and its onset, some deaf or hearing impaired people may communicate through speech only, and some, through a combination of sign language, finger-spelling, speech, and writing. Body language and facial expressions may be exaggerated, as they are also an important part of communication, especially for someone whose speech is not clear.

2. Use speech that seems strange. Hearing is critical to adequate speech and language development. People who are profoundly deaf may have never heard speech (not even their own). People who are deaf or hearing impaired may have never developed speaking abilities. Those who lost their hearing later in life may have lost their ability to speak clearly. Both problems may be caused by the absence of aural reinforcement. Also, all people use their ears as a monitoring system to regulate the quality and volume of their voices. This is not possible for people with a hearing loss, resulting in speech with inappropriate and strange pitch or volume control.

3. Carefully watch the lips of people to whom they are listening. Even if the deaf or hearing impaired individual has some hearing acuity, lipreading can substantially boost the accuracy with which he or she understands what is being said. Faint or distant speech is often aurally unintelligible to someone with a hearing loss, as are the words of someone who is speaking in a crowd of other people who are talking.

4. Exhibit a lack of vocabulary. Hearing children are far ahead of nonhearing children in both vocabulary and language development because, unlike their deaf counterparts, hearing children have been exposed to speech from the moment of birth and so have been able to develop a vocabulary merely from the incidental learning that accompanies listening.

5. Exhibit poor reading and writing skills. Children acquire language through their sense of hearing. This aurally developed language facility enables them to translate orally learned language into the

symbols of written communication. A child who does not know words has difficulty learning to read and write. Without special help, the average reading level of a deaf or hearing impaired child often does not increase beyond the third or fourth grade as the child reaches adulthood.

6.   Exhibit inconsistent behavior. This is because environmental factors influence a deaf or hearing impaired person's ability to hear the spoken word. For example, background noises can make hearing impossible for people who wear hearing aids. Also, those same people may hear what is being said but may not understand it because they are not familiar with some aspect of the spoken communication (e.g., idioms, unfamiliar words, and the like). Sometimes not hearing or not hearing well causes lack of attention or delays in responding to directions that have been given orally.

7.   Feel a sense of isolation. Many parents of deaf children do not know sign language so they cannot communicate with their own children. This lack of communication causes great isolation. Elderly people who lose their hearing also lose their ability to communicate. For many, sign language is too hard to learn, and writing is too tedious. The elderly person who is deaf may be facing a very lonely and isolated old age.

In even broader terms, as has been pointed out earlier, it is a myth that people who are deaf or hearing impaired are a homogeneous group. People who do not hear or who do not hear well differ from each other as definitely as all people do. It cannot be stressed enough that deafness does not affect a person's intellectual capacity, nor does it diminish in any way a person's ability to learn. A hearing loss merely cuts off people from acquiring and transmitting information in traditional oral/aural ways.

Needs of People Who Are Deaf or Hearing Impaired

A hearing disability generates needs. All of the needs listed below do not apply to every hearing impaired person.

Need for Communication Assistance. Many deaf or hearing impaired people are unable to participate in community activities or to use common services because of their inability to communicate via traditional modes. Because maintenance of independent functioning is, to a great extent, dependent on a person's ability to communicate, assistance in this area is critical.

Need for Employment Assistance. Many people who are deaf or hearing impaired complete their education without acquiring any specific job skills. Some enter the work force but later cannot continue in their customary work because of the onset of hearing difficulties. Employers are sometimes reluctant to hire people with a hearing loss or to keep them when a hearing loss occurs, often unaware of the capabilities of the deaf or hearing impaired. Employers should be encouraged to employ deaf and hearing impaired individuals and should be made aware of their success in the workplace as well as the many assistive aids available to compensate for deafness.

Need for Information Regarding Independent Living Skills. People who are deaf or hearing impaired, regardless of their age, require specific information about appropriate assistive devices that will facilitate their ability to move independently within society. In addition, they need easy access to these aids, training to use them, and help with other necessary independent living skills, not the least of which are strategies for communication.

Need to Combat Misinformation about Deafness. There are many myths and much misinformation about hearing loss. These must be combated by education, quality information, and quality referral. Information about deafness must be distributed and actively explained throughout a community. Until hearing people understand the difficulties encountered by a deaf or hearing impaired person who must function in a hearing world, all advances are too small and too slow.

Need for Information Provided through Advocacy. Although deaf or hearing impaired people are their own best advocates, there is need, also, for advocacy assistance from many types of organizations and from concerned hearing people who can communicate well enough in a hearing world to fight effectively the discrimination that faces deaf or hearing impaired people. Hearing advocates are a critical bridge between the hearing world and the silent world of the deaf or hearing impaired. Their most vital contribution is to provide interpreter services that ensure accurate understanding between deaf or hearing impaired individuals and hearing people.

Need to Identify Deafness Early. It is critical that a hearing loss be identified as soon as possible. Early identification of a hearing loss can result in the immediate use of assistive devices and the acquisition of adaptive living skills that will help prevent the isolation caused by a deaf or hearing impaired person's fear of approaching public institutions within the hearing world. Experiences of rejection by the hearing world often prevent people with hearing disabilities from approaching people and institutions whose companionship and services are the foundation of a fulfilled life. Paradoxically, deaf or hearing impaired people have a need for the services of public institutions, yet the very disability that causes the need is also what prevents them from remedying it.

Need for Literacy Training. Although there are many, many, exceptions, a large group of deaf or hearing impaired people never rises above a fifth-grade reading level. Regardless of innate ability, people who have a profound hearing loss (especially one that developed at birth or before the acquisition of language) experience difficulty with reading and writing because they have never heard the spoken word. The many conflicting educational theories and practices that now exist increase a deaf or hearing impaired person's inability to read or write in English because their use can lead to educational inconsistencies and confusion. There is a need for literacy classes that are designed to improve a deaf or hearing impaired person's basic communication skills in English.

Need for Special Education. A critical need at all levels is the availability of education tailored to enable people who are deaf or hearing impaired to take their places in the world. Whether for children or adults, the primary goal of any education/training system is to allow individuals to function in the mainstream of society.

Need to Coordinate Special Programs. Present programs geared toward deaf or hearing impaired people must be coordinated with each other as well as with any developed in the future. Lack of coordination causes redundancy and lack of access, keeping many people from receiving appropriate existing services.

Need to Enforce Present Regulations. Many people who are deaf or hearing impaired are not protected from discrimination because present regulations are not enforced. Specific attention should be given to changes in the educational system related to the education of people who are deaf or hearing impaired.

Need for Vocational Training. If people who are deaf or hearing impaired are to be independent and reach their fullest potential, specially delivered vocational training must be available.

Need for Increased Opportunities to Progress in a Career. Often, people who are deaf or hearing impaired have little problem securing initial employment. However, they may find that upward mobility is severely restricted or impossible. Barriers to upward mobility must be addressed through education (both employee and employer) and through incentive programs.

Need for Reduction of Barriers to Equal Access in the Private Sector. The 1973 Rehabilitation Act reduced barriers to equal access in the areas of business and government that received federal funds. Similar legislation is needed for the private sector. The American Disabilities Act, passed in the summer of 1990, helps.

Need for Interpreters. For many people who are deaf, interpreters are essential. There is a need for increased numbers of interpreters as well as for subsidies to help pay for their services when they are available.

Need for TDD Relay Services. Interstate Telecommunication Devices for the Deaf (TDD) Relay Services are needed to enable people who have a hearing loss to have the same opportunity as people who can hear to communicate effectively over the telephone. Many people who are deaf do not have private access to TDDs, nor are these communication devices available in enough quantity in critical areas such as care providing. A related service that is also necessary is public amplification devices for people who are hearing impaired.

Provision of Library Services to Deaf or Hearing Impaired People

Libraries are places where deaf or hearing impaired people can receive information in accessible formats, can pursue research, and can utilize recreational opportunities. To be able to use a library is a step toward complete integration into society in general.

The library and information needs of people who have a hearing loss do not differ to any great extent from those of people who hear. The mode of delivery, the format of materials, and the channels of communication are different. These must be modified in accordance with the degree and type of hearing loss. Sign language, lipreading, the written word, the printed word, pictures, amplification, and assistive aids are all helpful. To determine which is most appropriate, librarians must learn as much as possible about the deaf or hearing impaired community.

A successful approach to meeting the needs of people who are deaf or hearing impaired is to identify their needs through a series of planned meetings with library staff. As needs are cooperatively identified, the library staff and the deaf community can determine who should meet these needs, how much funding is required, how the funds can be secured, when they will be available, and how long it will take to realize the desired results.

In the delivery of library programs to fill the needs of people who have hearing difficulties, the following questions can be asked: Are these needs currently being met by any other agencies in the community? Which agencies should concentrate funds, energies, and personnel resources to meet these needs? Is the current level of funding among the agencies adequate to provide the full range of activities at the appropriate level and in the appropriate modes of communication? If not, how much additional funding is required to meet the diverse needs of people who do not hear at all or do not hear well?

Libraries and librarians can provide a variety of services to the deaf or hearing impaired.

Gaining Employment. Librarians can play a vital role in the process of identifying and developing employment opportunities for people with a hearing loss.

Obtaining Special Education. Librarians are in a unique position to directly provide, sponsor, or coordinate educational programs. There is a need for programs for deaf or hearing impaired people at all ages and at all levels of education. Literacy training is especially important for the 30 percent of the deaf population that is illiterate.

Facilitating Creativity. Librarians can assist in obtaining recognition of artists, authors, performers, and other creative individuals who have a hearing loss.

Promoting Technology. With the installation and use of communication aids, including Telecommunication Devices for the Deaf (TDD), librarians not only demonstrate the value of the technology but also can serve as communicators from deaf or hearing impaired people to agencies without TDDs.

Providing Recreational Opportunities. Libraries need to become as great a part of the recreational pursuits of people who have a hearing loss as they are of those of the entire general public.

Becoming Accessible. By being totally accessible to people who are deaf or hearing impaired, libraries can provide a model for others.

Communicating. Librarians should know the various modes of communication people with a hearing loss use and develop services accordingly. To reiterate, deaf and hearing impaired people may communicate through the use of:

- Sign language. Manual communication (sign language) is used by many people who are deaf as an effective means of communication. Library staff members need to be able to understand the sign language used and to be fairly fluent in it themselves. Sign language varies from the use of the manual alphabet to the use of American Sign Language (ASL), which is based on concepts rather than on letters. To be fluent in manual communication, library staff members must learn the language and use it to retain their fluency.
- Lipreading. Many people who are deaf read lips rather than sign or use another manual means of communication. Many have understandable speech. While lipreading is excellent for some people, its use by others can cause a great loss in the transmission and receipt of information. For greatest success, information should be shared while people face each other and speak in a normal, not exaggerated, mode. Also, the person speaking should face into the light.

- Writing. Communication can take place through the written word. Because a person who is deaf may not have a large vocabulary, the written communication should be straightforward in clear, short sentences. It must also be legible to people who may not be familiar with more than one style of handwriting.
- Hearing aids and other auditory aids. Many people who become deaf after having reached adulthood may rely on hearing aids as a method of communication. In such instances it is important that voices be kept at a normal level and that pronunciation be clear but not exaggerated. Auditory aids that amplify sound will help some hearing impaired people enjoy general public programs.
- Interpreters. Use of a third person is another means of communication. An interpreter translates speech into sign language for the person who is deaf and then translates sign language into speech for the hearing person.
- TDDs and telephone amplification devices. Deaf and hearing impaired persons increasingly are making use of the telephone by means of a telecommunication device for the deaf (TDD). Because it is difficult and sometimes impossible for deaf or hearing impaired individuals to use the telephone, TDDs must be available for access to all telephone services available to the general public. In the case of many hearing impaired people, amplification of tone on a regular telephone will suffice and should be explored.
- Directional and informational signs. Communication can be greatly enhanced by directional and informational signs that use the international code as well as English. It should be noted that international code symbols help all people who do not read English (not just deaf or hearing impaired people). Because of the limited vocabulary of many people who are deaf or hearing impaired, the language of all signs must be simple, clear, and direct.

Provision of Special Materials. Because reading skills vary considerably among deaf or hearing impaired people, high interest/low vocabulary reading materials are often needed. Often, the average reading level for people who are deaf is very low (about fifth grade level); visual and heavily illustrated print materials are a necessity. Transparencies, picture story sets, photo-motion sets, games, and captioned films are popular. Television sets with decoders enable people who have a hearing loss to enjoy closed-captioned television, which is also appreciated.

People who are deaf or hearing impaired need up-to-date information on deafness and hearing impairments. This includes medical, legal, and educational materials. Reading materials that focus on the cultural and life experiences of people who do not hear well are also most important. The bibliotherapeutic benefits of these materials cannot be overemphasized. The needs of family members should also be addressed. When deafness occurs at birth or in early childhood, materials about deafness should be available for the child's parents and family, all of whom may be dealing with deafness for the first time. They need information that will allow them to have appropriate expectations and that will give them the ability to judge services and facilities accurately. When hearing loss occurs during adulthood, family members require information to help them deal with the changed circumstances in communication and the stresses that inevitably occur as they try to preserve relationships.

Provision of Meeting Places. Many organizations exist for people who are deaf or hearing impaired. There is a need, which the library can easily fill, for suitable meeting places equipped with auditory aids and appropriate lighting to facilitate the deaf or hearing impaired person's dependence upon lipreading and interpreters.

Marketing. Libraries are not usually a part of the life of people with a long history of hearing loss. This is because the essence of librarianship is communication, the area in which deaf or hearing impaired people have the most difficulty. Because libraries and librarians represent institutions that have not traditionally been accessible to people with a hearing loss, they are often avoided by deaf or hearing impaired people. A well-constructed marketing program is critical to let people with a hearing loss know that the library has much to offer. Such a project requires, initially, a concentrated focus on the deaf community. Deaf or hearing impaired people are the only reliable sources for identifying the needs of their population group. It is vital that the specific needs of each deaf community within a library's population group be fully identified.

Once a program is in place and has had a reasonable time to prove itself, it must be evaluated by the deaf community. The library staff can evaluate the cost and the performance, but only the deaf community can determine if the program accomplishes its purpose.

It should again be emphasized that, to provide appropriate library services for deaf and hearing impaired people, librarians must understand their needs. This can be accomplished best by working with deaf or hearing impaired people and especially by employing them. Although many libraries have people who are deaf or hearing impaired on their staffs, the number is not as yet large enough to ensure that people who have a hearing loss work meaningfully together with those who do not.

Agencies That Can Provide Information about Library Service to People Who Are Deaf or Hearing Impaired

While there are many sources of information relating to deafness and hearing impairment in general, the following are important agencies that can provide much help.

Alexander Graham Bell Association for the Deaf, Inc.
3417 Volta Place NW
Washington, DC 20007

The association is devoted to finding more effective ways of teaching people who are deaf or hearing impaired. It provides information concerning deafness, especially oralism and children's rights. The association also provides publications and information on training and development of oral interpreters.

American Society for Deaf Children (formerly International
Association of Parents of the Deaf)
814 Thayer Avenue
Silver Spring, Maryland 20910

The society provides information and support to parents and families with children who are deaf or hearing impaired.

Captioned Films for the Deaf
5000 Park Street, N.
St. Petersburg, FL 33709

This network of libraries operates under federal funding to distribute films relating to deafness to groups of people who are deaf and to institutions and organizations serving people who are deaf.

Friends of Libraries for Deaf Action
PO Box 50045
Washington, DC 20004-0045

The friends provide information about library service to people who are deaf or hearing impaired. The group provides excellent material relating to Deaf Heritage Month. It issues a useful publication known as the *Red Notebook*.

Helen Keller National Center for Deaf-Blind Youths and Adults
111 Middle Neck Road
Sands Point, NY 11050

This national organization is a source of much information on library service to people who are deaf and blind. It provides evaluation and rehabilitation training for deaf-blind youths and adults and compiles the *Directory of Agencies Serving Deaf/Blind*.

Gallaudet University
800 Florida Avenue, NE
Washington, DC 20002

The library in this university, as well as the entire university, can provide a wealth of information. Gallaudet is the only liberal arts university in the world for people who are deaf. Among the materials that the university produces are lists of captioned videotapes currently available on the market. The university publishes *Gallaudet Today*.

Library Service to the Deaf Forum
American Library Association
50 East Huron Street
Chicago, IL 60611

A unit of the American Library Association's Division of the Association of Specialized and Cooperative Library Agencies, this group, among its other activities, operates a clearinghouse for information and provides services for the purpose of assisting libraries to develop collections and programs related to deafness.

The National Association for Hearing and Speech Action
10801 Rockville Pike
Rockville, MD 20852

In addition to providing information regarding nonhearing people, the association provides information about TDDs.

National Association of the Deaf
814 Thayer Avenue
Silver Spring, MD 20910

This national consumer association of people from the deaf community covers broad issues that affect the lives of people who are deaf or hearing impaired. It functions as a clearinghouse for information on total communication. The association publishes *NAD Broadcaster* and *Deaf American*.

National Captioning Institute, Inc.
5203 Leesburg Pike
Falls Church, VA 22041

This organization provides information on closed-captioning. It also provides information lists of closed-captioned material available on the market. Its primary goal is to make captioned television available to every deaf or hearing impaired person who wants it.

National Technical Institute for the Deaf
1 Lomb Memorial Drive
Rochester, NY 14621

The institute provides information on deafness as well as resources for the education of deaf professionals.

The President's Committee on Employment of People with Disabilities
1111 20th Street, NW
Washington, DC 20036

This committee provides advice and information to facilitate development of maximum employment opportunities for people who are physically disabled, mentally ill, or retarded. It publishes *Worklife: A Publication on Employment and People with Disabilities*.

Self-Help for Hard of Hearing People, Inc.
7800 Wisconsin Avenue
Bethesda, MD 20814

With chapters throughout the United States, this self-help group publishes *Shhh Journal*. Because it is a self-help organization, attendance at meetings is most valuable.

The organizations listed above are supplemented and sometimes surpassed by service clubs as resources for information about services for people who are deaf or hearing impaired. Among the more well known service clubs are:

Lions Clubs International
300 22d Street
Oak Brook, IL 60521

A major goal of the Lions Clubs is to provide resources and information related to deafness. Of special mention is the work that this club has done to purchase TDDs for libraries. The group also has information about closed-captioning for television.

Pilot International
PO Box 4844
244 College Street
Macon, GA 31213-0599

Founded with the goal of achieving full citizenship for people with disabilities, the organization has, on the local level, provided assistive equipment for the deaf to libraries. Each year, a disabled professional person of the year is selected. In some instances, the person receiving the award has had a hearing loss.

Quota International
1420 21st Street NW
Washington, DC 20036

Through its project, "Shatter Silence," members of Quota International have been involved with libraries and have benefited deaf or hearing impaired people through their work. Service to people with hearing losses and difficulties with speech has, since 1964, been a major concern of the Quota Club.

Sertoma International
1912 E. Meyer Boulevard
Kansas City, MO 64132-1174

Through its "Local Action" program, the foundation provides a direct link to those who have problems in communication.

Zonta International
557 W. Randolph Street
Chicago, IL 60606

This service organization promotes closed-captioned television programs for people with a hearing loss.

References

About Barriers. 1982. Washington, D.C.: Architectural and Transportation Barriers Compliance Board.

"Americans with Disabilities Act." 1990. *Information from Heath* 9 (Fall): 1, 3, 10.

Biehl, J. 1984. *Helping the Deaf Patron in the Library*. Canton, Ohio: Stark County District Library.

Boone, S., and G. A. Long, eds. 1988. *Enhancing the Employability of Deaf Persons: Model Interventions*. Springfield, Ill.: Charles C. Thomas.

Bowe, F. 1986. *Changing the Rules*. Silver Spring, Md.: T. J. Publishers.

Bowe, F. 1984. *Personal Computers and Special Needs*. Berkeley, Calif.: SYBEX.

Bunch, G. O. 1987. *The Curriculum and the Hearing-Impaired Student: Theoretical and Practical Considerations*. Boston: Little, Brown.

"Cooperation Improves Library Service to the Blind and Deaf." 1987. *Link-Up* 42 (January): 1-28.

Crossroads. July 1986. International edition 1: entire issue.

Dalton, P. I. 1990. "Awards Programs as Incentives for the Employment of People with Disabilities." *Library Personnel News* 4 (Summer): 43-44.

_____. 1985. *Library Service to the Deaf and Hearing Impaired*. Phoenix: Oryx Press.

_____. 1990. "1990s Agenda: Full Employment for All." *Library Personnel News* 4 (Summer): 45-46.

_____. 1990. "Productivity, Not Paternalism." *Library Personnel News* 4 (Summer):42-43.

_____. 1985. "Video and Library Service to the Deaf–United States." In *Video in Libraries, an International Perspective*, edited by P. McNally, 69-81. The Hague, Netherlands: Nederlands Bibliotheek en Lektur Centrum.

Farb, A. B. 1990. "Bush Signs ADA Bill." *NAD Broadcaster* 12 (August/September): 1-2.

Freeland, A. 1989. *Deafness: The Facts*. New York: Oxford University Press.

Gannon, J. R. 1981. *Deaf Heritage: A Narrative History of Deaf in America*. Silver Spring, Md.: National Association of the Deaf.

Garretson, M. D., ed. 1990. "Communication Issues among Deaf People." *A Deaf American Notebook* 40: 1-138.

Hagemeyer, A. September 1981. "Library Service to the Deaf and Outreach Programs for the Deaf." *Illinois Libraries* 63, no. 7: 530-35.

"Hard of Hearing Students on Campus." 1990. *Information from Heath* 9 (Fall): 1, 4-5.

Johnstone, M. 1986. "Meeting Students' Needs." *Gallaudet Today* 16 (Winter): 6-9.

Jones, D. E. 1989. "Serving Everyone: Government Documents to Serve the Physically Handicapped." *Illinois Libraries*, November, 466-71.

Kaplan, H. 1985. "Hearing Loss in Later Life." *Shhh* 6 (May/June): 7-8, 21.

Karr, A. R. 1990. "Disabled Rights Bill Inspires Hope, Fear." *Wall Street Journal*, 21 May, 1, 2.

Lovejoy, E. 1990. *Portraits of Library Service to People with Disabilities*. Boston: G. K. Hall.

Masters, S. R. n.d. *What! A Hearing Impaired Child in My Class?* Pittsford, N.Y.: Susan R. Masters.

Moon, V. 1986. *Library Services for People with Disabilities*. Sydney, Australia: State Library of New South Wales.

"The Most Important Law So Far: Americans with Disabilities Act of 1989." 1989. *AADC News*, Summer, 1, 8.

National Institute of Neurological Diseases and Stroke. 1982 *Hearing Loss: Hope through Research*. Bethesda, Md.: National Institutes of Health.

National Library of Australia. 1985. *Library Services to Deaf and Hearing Impaired People: A Selected Bibliography*. Canberra: National Library of Australia.

Needham, W. L., and G. Jahoda. 1983. *Improving Library Service to Physically Disabled Persons*. Littleton, Colo.: Libraries Unlimited.

New York Library Association. Roundtable for Libraries Serving Special Populations. 1987. *Guidelines for Libraries Serving Persons with a Hearing or Visual Impairment*. Albany: New York Library Association.

Noah, T. 1990. "Legislation Will Give Disabled People Greater Leverage to Gain Access to Jobs." *Wall Street Journal*, 21 May, 1, 4.

Opening Doors for Closed Ears: Conference on Library Services for Deaf and Hearing Impaired People. 1988. Sydney, Australia: State Library of New South Wales.

Padden, C., and T. Humphries. 1988. *Deaf in America: Voices from a Culture*. Cambridge: Harvard University Press.

The President's Committee on Employment of People with Disabilities. 1989. *Annual Work Plan, 1989*. Washington, D.C.: The Committee.

"The President's Committee Meeting and ADA: A Special Report." 1990. *Worklife* 5 (Summer): 17-29.

The Red Notebook and Supplements. 1989. Washington, D.C.: Friends of Libraries for Deaf Action.

"Reflections after 10 Years: PL 94-142 and Deafness." 1986. *Gallaudet Today* 16 (Winter): 3-6.

Rivlin, A. M., and J. M. Wiener. 1988. *Caring for the Disabled Elderly: Who Will Pay?* Washington, D.C.: The Brookings Institution.

Serving Deaf Students in Academic Libraries. 1983. Two audio cassettes. Chicago, Ill.: American Library Association.

Stone, H. 1990. "Americans with Disabilities Act Becomes Law!" *Southwest Focus* 2 (July/August): 1, 9, 14, 15.

Summary of Existing Legislation Affecting People with Disabilities. 1987. Washington, D.C.: Department of Education, Office of Special Education and Rehabilitative Services, Clearinghouse on the Handicapped.

Sundstrom, S. C. 1983. *Understanding Hearing Loss and What Can Be Done to Help*. Danville, Ill.: Interstate Printers and Publishers.

TDD Library Newsletter. 1986-89. Trenton: New Jersey State Library, selected issues.

Thomas, J. L., and C. H. Thomas. 1982. *Library Services for the Handicapped Adult*. Phoenix: Oryx Press.

Tips You Can Use When Communicating with Deaf People. 1980. Rochester, N.Y.: National Technical Institute for the Deaf, Rochester Institute of Technology.

Velleman, R. A. 1990. *Meeting the Needs of People with Disabilities: A Guide for Librarians, Educators, and Other Service Professionals*. Phoenix: Oryx Press.

Weir, G., and C. Law. 1986. *Quiet, Please! Deaf People Are Coming: How to Make Libraries Accessible for People with a Hearing Impairment*. Canberra: National Library of Australia.

Wright, K., and J. F. Davie. 1990. *Library Manager's Guide to Hiring and Serving Disabled Persons*. Jefferson, N.C.: McFarland and Co.

Appendix: Sensitizing Activities for Librarians

Many of the sensitizing activities contained in this appendix are reprinted with permission from various sources. Each of the mentioned sources can provide valuable additional information and is recommended as supplemental reading.

Sensitizing Activity for Visual Impairment

The following page is reprinted with permission of the Association on Handicapped Student Service Programs in Postsecondary Education (AHSSPPE). It is taken from their publication, AHSSPPE Inservice Education Kit *(1988).*

The print on the following page approximates the clarity with which a visually impaired person might see different sizes of type. It is an illustration of the value of large type because the larger the type, the easier it is for a visually impaired person to read without the aid of an assistive device.

Totally blind patrons will read via their ears. The best example of this type of reading is playing a taped book for the audience.

8 Point Type

Few parents realize that during the progress of these diseases the eyes of the patient may develop serious ulcers or other dangerous conditions, which, unless skilfully treated, may leave a white film over the "sight" of the eye

10 Point Type

Few parents realize that during the progress of these diseases the eyes of the patient may develop serious ulcers or other dangerous conditions, which, unless skilfully treated,

12 Point Type

Few parents realize that during the progress of these diseases the eyes of the patient may develop serious ulcers or other dangerous conditions, which, unless

14 Point Type

Few parents realize that during the progress of these diseases the eyes of the patient

18 Point Type

Few parents realize that during the progress of these diseases the

24 Point Type

Few parents realize that during the progress of these

30 Point Type

Few parents realize that during the prog-

Sensitizing Activities for Learning Disabilities

The following activities are reprinted with permission of the Association on Handicapped Student Service Programs in Postsecondary Education (AHSSPPE). They are taken from their publication, AHSSPPE Inservice Education Kit *(1988).*

Activity One

One way to simulate the problems that patrons with motor coordination (eye-hand) problems may experience is to use the image of a star that follows this text. Put the paper with the star on the table in front of each person. Have each of the audience members hold a small mirror about 12 inches above the star so that they can see the reflection of the star in the mirror, but not the star itself. Now, while looking at the reflection of the star have the audience members trace over the star on the paper without looking at the paper. You will find that the lines drawn will not at all follow the lines already on the paper. People will have tremendous problems with direction, changing direction at each of the points, and with staying on the lines that are already there. Some people will do better than others, simulating the varying degrees to which a learning disabled person may be affected by the disability. Note: It is important that the mirror be held above the star so that the tracers have to look up at the mirror and cannot see the star on the paper.

Activity Two

On the page following the star is a printed passage that simulates some of the problems a dyslexic patron might have reading. Note that some words are backwards, some letters are transposed, and the transpositions are not always the same, making it very difficult for someone with dyslexia to compensate for the problem.

Have the audience read this passage out loud. You will find that they will have difficulty. Some will be better at reading this than others. Again, this simulates the varying degrees to which a patron might be affected by dyslexia.

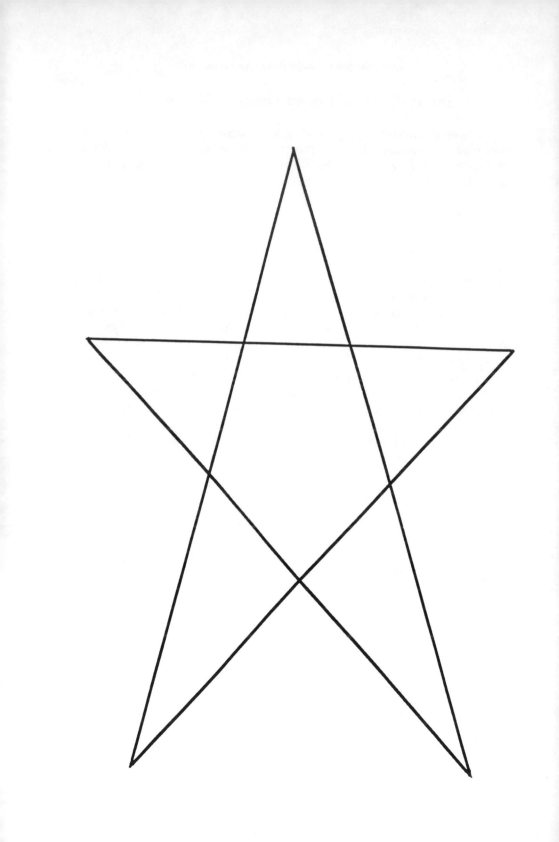

In mobern soceity, an inbivibual's ytiliba to be self-sufficient is usually encouraqed from childhood. By eht tine we are adults, we are uspposed to have learmed to debend upon ourselves, to de as puick on the ward as the next persom and to be ready to dolh our own in a more or less ilesoht world.

Inbeqenbence is also comsidered a civic virtue, for self-relaicne means pulling your own thgiew, paying your taxes and not deing a durben on your hard-rpsseed fellow countrymcn. The enphasis in almost lla bencial rehabilitation is to retrain the disblaed person for productive work. If siht qroves unfeasible, they nay de considered useless and left to hsiugnal apart from the naimstrean.

This atttiued quts tremendous pressure no the disabled norimyiit. Trying to keep threi self-respect im a society that equates inbeqenbemce with physical well-being nakes an already tluciffid situation almost elbarelotni, for the hamdicaqqed person is generally persauded to think the sane way. Such emphasisover on paying ome's yaw seems to leave disabled qeoqle with only wot alternatives - - to knock themselves uot trying to etepmoc om able-ddiebo terms or ot opt out entirely. This limited ccoihe would mot apply if soceity acknowledged other teriairc of worth.

It's inportamt to realize that on individual can really tsixe alone. Im a civilized society ew are all interbeqendent. And, at best, physical deinpendence is variable. Able-bodied or not, everyome experiences sdoirep of debenqence: illness and dlo age are undiscrinimating. Moral inqebendence, on the other hand, is elbitcurtsedni.

Adapted from Glorya Hale, ed., *The Source Book for the Disabled* (New York: Paddington Press, 1979), 40-41.

Sensitizing Activities for Hearing Impairment and Deafness

The sign language demonstration on the following pages, used in activity one, is adapted from the Association on Handicapped Student Service Programs in Postsecondary Education Inservice Education Kit *(1988). Illustrations for the sign language demonstration were contributed by Carolyn R. Sturtevant.*

The examples of poor syntactic structure used in activity two are from Frederick N. Martin's Pediatric Audiology *(Englewood Cliffs, N.J.: Prentice-Hall, 1978).*

Activity One

The presenter will first make a blackboard drawing or a chart of the page entitled "Drawing for Chalkboard or Flipchart for Signing Demonstration." The presenter will then mouth (without vocalizing) the script provided on the sheet entitled "Chalkboard or Flipchart Script." As the presenter mouths the words, the presenter will point to the appropriate symbol on the board (i.e., the first circle with a line through it on the board is "this is a wug," the second square with a line through it on the board is "this is a wag," etc.). After mouthing the script, the presenter will motion for an audience member to come up and answer some questions, which the presenter will also mouth. The questions are on the sheet entitled "Questions for Sign Language Demonstration." You will find that the person being asked the questions will probably be totally confused and will not be able to even understand your mouthed questions.

After this, the presenter will again present the script from the beginning of the sign language demonstration script; only this time he or she will sign the mouthed words and point to the figures on the board. The signs for the script are under the words on the "Sign Language Demonstration Script." (The signs provided are approximations of how the script might be signed.)

Now, the presenter will call a person from the audience to answer the questions asked earlier. This time, the person asked to come up and answer questions will be asked with a combination of mouthing and signing. (Refer to the sheet titled "Questions for Sign Language Demonstration, with signs.") You will find that this time, the person asked to answer the questions will actually be able to answer a good portion of the questions.

The exercise demonstrates the value of sign language. It also demonstrates the difficulties of lipreading.

Note: The same script is used for both presentations of the exercise. The first time, the words are only mouthed–no voicing is used so the audience must rely on lipreading. When a member of the audience comes up to try to answer the questions, score them on a chalkboard or overhead as "correct" and "incorrect" for all to see. The second time through, the exercise and the questions are presented by mouthing the script, pointing to the figures on the board, and using sign but still not using voice. To do this, the script must be committed to memory. Again, score the participant responses as correct and incorrect so that all can see how much better one can do with signing added in.

Drawing for Chalkboard or Flipchart for Signing Demonstration

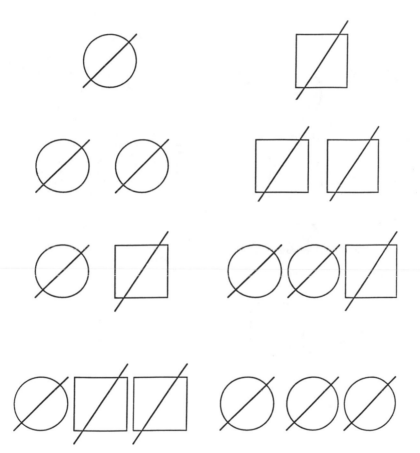

Chalkboard or Flipchart Script

THIS IS A WUG.

THIS IS A WAG.

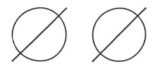

THIS WUG HAS A FRIEND.   IT IS ANOTHER WUG.

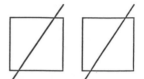

HERE WE HAVE TWO WAGS TOGETHER.
THIS WAG HAS A FRIEND.
IT IS ANOTHER WAG.
HERE WE HAVE TWO WAGS TOGETHER.

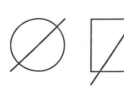

THIS WUG HAS A FRIEND.   HIS FRIEND IS A WAG.

HERE WE HAVE A WUG AND A WAG TOGETHER.

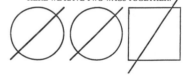

THIS TIME I HAVE TWO WUGS BUT ONLY ONE WAG.
HERE ARE TWO WUGS AND ONE WAG TOGETHER.

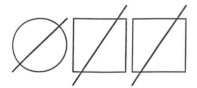

NOW I HAVE TWO WAGS BUT ONLY ONE WUG.

HERE ARE TWO WAGS AND ONE WUG TOGETHER.

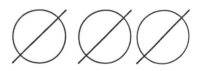

WHAT DO I HAVE HERE?
THREE WUGS.
HERE ARE THREE WUGS TOGETHER.

Questions for Sign Language Demonstration

SHOW ME A WUG.

SHOW ME A WAG.

SHOW ME TWO WAGS TOGETHER.

SHOW ME TWO WUGS TOGETHER.

SHOW ME THREE WUGS TOGETHER.

SHOW ME TWO WUGS AND ONE WAG.

THANK YOU. YOU CAN SIT DOWN.

Sign Language Demonstration Script

THIS   IS   A   WUG.   THIS   IS   A   WAG.

 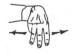

THIS WUG HAS A FRIEND. IT IS ANOTHER WUG.

HERE   WE   HAVE   TWO   WAGS   TOGETHER.

THIS   WAG   HAS   A   FRIEND.

IT IS ANOTHER WAG.

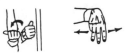

HERE WE HAVE TWO WAGS TOGETHER.

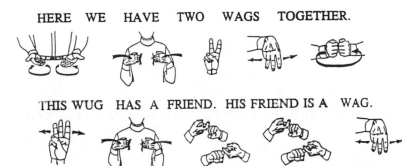

THIS WUG HAS A FRIEND. HIS FRIEND IS A WAG.

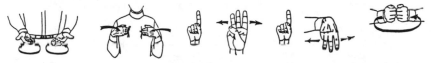

HERE WE HAVE A WUG AND A WAG TOGETHER.

THIS   TIME,   I   HAVE   TWO   WUGS,

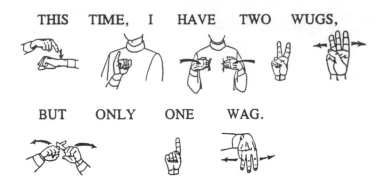

BUT   ONLY   ONE   WAG.

HERE ARE TWO WUGS AND ONE WAG TOGETHER.

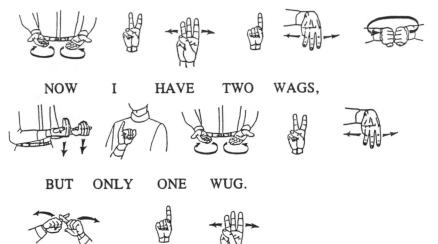

NOW   I   HAVE   TWO   WAGS,

BUT   ONLY   ONE   WUG.

HERE ARE TWO WAGS AND ONE WUG TOGETHER.

   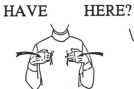 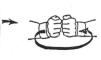

WHAT   DO   I   HAVE   HERE?

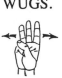

THREE   WUGS.

HERE   ARE   THREE   WUGS   TOGETHER.

87

Questions for Sign Language Demonstration, with Signs

NOW IT'S YOUR TURN. WILL YOU COME UP HERE?

For this line, just point to a person, and gesture for him/her to come up.

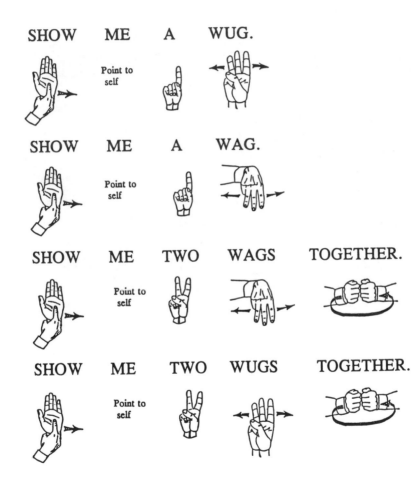

SHOW   ME   THREE   WUGS   TOGETHER.

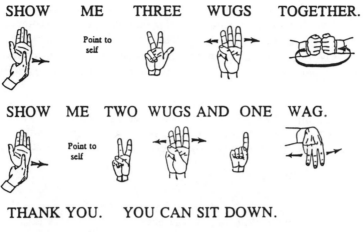

SHOW   ME   TWO   WUGS AND   ONE   WAG.

THANK YOU.   YOU CAN SIT DOWN.

Gesture for the participant to sit down.

Activity Two

An effective way to demonstrate the written communication difficulties of individuals who have been deaf before acquiring language and its structure is to provide some samples of their writing. The frustration of knowing what one wants to say but not being understood because of poor syntactic structures can be seen quite well in these examples from Martin's *Pediatric Audiology:*

> The man pull many her fish. He see one large fish. The boy saw many, many her fish and turtle. The man saw two red fish. He will see not out more and fish. The boy is sorry. (10-year-old female, born deaf).

> The girl help to dog eat. The children had talk. The family went to trip. The boy saw to dog. A boy was happy to met dog. A dog want to in car. Our family leave to on trip. Our family arrived to rest in park. The two boy played to ball or with the dog. Some Children was hungry. A woman cooked to the hamburg. A girl want to eat. (14-year-old male, born deaf).

> Mrs. Gloria made some sandwich and other some any food and drink. A little girl got a sandwich. She give a dog eat a cheese and ham sandwich. She brother Bill tooked I gave basketball for bring park. and father got a bat and ball. A Family arrived father is car. He drive car It is on. Happen Bill saw a dog walked on the sidewalk. He told father, He said stop. He say what. I saw may a dog. Open a door. Bill jumped on the side walk. He love him dog. He laught them Now We went to trip for park. About 1:30 oclock. Mrs. Gloria cooked hamburger and other sandwich. Father son Bill played baseball. A dog running to Bill because a dog get a ball. but we have good time for park. (18-year-old male, born deaf).

Sensitizing Activity for Mental Retardation

It is difficult to simulate the experience of mental retardation. The following exercise, although not ideal, does demonstrate some of the reactions that people who cannot do the same work as their peers might have. Following are two copies of a math test. One is in English; the other is in Chinese. The presenter should hand the test out to the audience, face down, and direct the audience not to turn the test over until told. The presenter should pass out some tests in Chinese and the majority of the tests in English. Tell the audience that the test is an easy one, so they will be given one minute to finish it. Direct them to raise their hands when they have completed the test.

You will notice a variety of responses around the room. Some of the participants who were given the Chinese test will be looking around at the other participants, some will be laughing, some will look confused, and some will raise their hands, even though they have not even started the assignment.

After the minute is over, the presenter should discuss the reactions of the people who were given the Chinese version. Their reactions are similar to the reactions of some mentally retarded individuals. They are embarrassed not to be able to do the same work as their peers, they sometimes act inappropriately because of their inability to keep up, and they sometimes pretend to have accomplished the task in order not to stand out.

Math Test

3 + 5 =   6 + 1 =   4 + 2 =

10 - 8 =   9 - 3 =   4 - 0 =

Chinese Math Test

叁加伍. 陆加壹. 肆加贰

拾加捌 玖减叁. 肆减零

Annotated Bibliography

RASHELLE S. KARP

This bibliography lists only those materials that the writer feels would be especially useful for librarians needing practical, easily applicable information. The citations are listed under subject headings to facilitate more direct access.

Accessibility

Conn, D. R., and B. McCallum. 1982. "Design for Accessibility." *Canadian Library Journal* 39 (June): 119-25.
    In this guide to designing and altering libraries to meet the needs of handicapped patrons, suggestions are given regarding site design, entryways, lighting, stairs and elevators, height of shelves, equipment, and furniture.

Duncan, J., comp. 1977. "Environment Modifications for the Visually Impaired: A Handbook." *Journal of Visual Impairment and Blindness* 71 (December): 442-55.
    Although older, the discussion of kinds and sources of information that can be used in planning environmental modifications to accommodate visually impaired patrons is still useful.

Kamisar, H. 1979. "Signs for the Handicapped Patron." In *Sign Systems for Libraries: Solving the Wayfinding Problem*, edited by Dorothy Pollett and Peter C. Haskell, 99-103. New York: Bowker.

This provides an excellent checklist of major design elements that must be considered when developing a total guidance system.

Keys, C. 1983. *Accessibility: Designing Buildings for the Needs of Handicapped Persons.* Washington, D.C.: National Library Service for the Blind and Physically Handicapped, Library of Congress.

This annotated bibliography lists books, articles, reports, and films on barrier-free design for disabled persons. With a few exceptions, all listed items have been published after 1978.

Needham, W. L., and G. Jahoda. 1983. *Improving Library Service to Physically Disabled Persons.* Littleton, Colo.: Libraries Unlimited.

This excellent checklist has been designed to allow librarians in all types of libraries to determine how to improve the accessibility of their library facilities and services. The book is now out of print, but the core of the checklist can also be found in Needham and Jahoda's "Academic Library Service to Handicapped Students" (*Journal of Academic Librarianship*, November 1977, 273-79).

Steinfeld, E. 1979. *Access to the Built Environment: A Review of Literature.* Washington, D.C.: U.S. Department of Housing and Urban Development, Office of Policy Development and Research.

Although older, the discussions here regarding access as a civil right, codes and regulations pertaining to accessibility, and the scope of barrier-free design, in addition to the bibliographies at the ends of the chapters, are still useful.

Agencies

Learning Disabilities: National Information and Advocacy Organizations. 1990. Washington, D.C.: National Library Service for the Blind and Physically Handicapped, Library of Congress.

This reference circular provides information about national organizations that serve as information clearinghouses or referral agencies or that act as advocacy organizations.

"Libraries for the Blind and Physically Handicapped." In *American Library Directory.* Published annually. New York: R.R. Bowker Co.

The *American Library Directory* provides a listing of the regional and subregional libraries of the Library of Congress National Library Service for the Blind and Physically Handicapped located throughout the country. This list is also published in other separately sold resources. If the library already has a standing order for the *American Library Directory*, other resources may not need to be purchased.

"Libraries Serving the Deaf and Hearing Impaired." In *American Library Directory*. Published annually. New York: R.R. Bowker Co.

This is a selective listing of libraries in the United States that provide TTY or TDD reference service. The listing serves as a special index to the directory.

Library Resources for the Blind and Physically Handicapped. A Directory of Division of the Blind and Physically Handicapped Network Libraries and Machine Lending Agencies. Published annually. Washington, D.C.: National Library Service for the Blind and Physically Handicapped, Library of Congress.

This is a directory of NLS network libraries and machine-lending agencies in the United States. The addresses listed here duplicate in part the addresses in the *American Library Directory*. However, the resource is free, and some of the machine-lending agencies listed here are not listed in the *American Library Directory*.

Majeska, M. L. 1988. *Talking Books: Pioneering and Beyond*. Washington, D.C.: National Library Service for the Blind and Physically Handicapped, Library of Congress.

In this excellent monograph, the history of the NLS talking-book program is detailed from 1932 through 1988. This, along with the NLS bulletin *News* (issued every two months), provides a historical and continuing accounting of the services and innovations of the NLS.

Senkevitch, J. J. 1979. "Toward a National Rehabilitation Data Base." *ASIS Bulletin* 5 (April): 14-15.

This brief discussion of the history, goals, and current activities of NARIC (National Rehabilitation Information Center) is useful for understanding the workings of an important information center.

Aids and Appliances

Bolnick, D., and B. C. Johnson. 1989. "Audiocassette Repair." *Library Journal* 114 (15 November): 43-46.

This has extremely detailed but clear instructions for repairing audio cassettes.

Chandler, J. G. 1979. "Voice Indexing of Tape Records." *Journal of Visual Impairment and Blindness* 73 (May): 191-92.
    The voice-indexing process by which individuals can audibly index their own cassette tapes, the types of equipment needed, and its unlimited possibilities for use are described.

Cushman, R. 1980. "The Kurzweil Reading Machine." *Wilson Library Bulletin* 54 (January): 311-15.
    Cushman describes how the Kurzweil machine works and how it may be used.

Edwards, S. 1989. "Computer Technology and the Physically Disabled." *OCLC Micro* 5 (October): 22-23, 25.
    Computer companies that manufacture software and hardware for physically disabled people are described, as are organizations that can provide information about the software and hardware.

_____. 1989. "Microcomputers and the Visually Impaired (Low-Vision to No-Vision)." *OCLC Micro* 5 (December): 20-21, 25-26.
    Software packages that magnify computer screen output or change print output into speech are identified and described.

Gillikin, D. P. 1989. "Customizing Database Searching for the Visually Impaired." *Database Searcher* 5 (October): 20-24.
    Special equipment and programming that allow visually impaired end users to access online bibliographic utilities are described.

Haynes, D. E. 1989. "The Switch Library: New Service in Rehabilitation Librarianship." *Bulletin of the Medical Library Association* 77 (January): 15-18.
    Microswitches allow "centralized control of many features of adapted residential environments" (i.e., heating, cooling, lights) and should be made available via library circulating collections to physically disabled individuals.

Howell, R. 1989. "Some Issues Related to Technological Intervention with Disabled Learners: Cues for Instructional Designers." *Ohio Media Spectrum* 41 (Fall): 50-53.
    Howell raises questions about technology, which is often developed *for* disabled individuals but is not developed with their input. A plan for including disabled individuals in the creative process of designing new technology is presented.

Jahoda, G., and E. A. Johnson. 1987. "The Use of the Kurzweil Reading Machine in Academic Libraries." *Journal of Academic Librarianship* 13 (May): 99-101, 103.

A survey of 50 academic libraries indicates that Kurzweil reading machines are underutilized. Lengthy training sessions, the need for perseverance, poor locations, and scheduling problems are suggested as contributing causes to lack of popularity. Some increase in use could be gained by greater assistance from librarians in providing relevant documents.

Johnson, R. M. 1986. "Kurzweil Reading Machine: Problems and Solutions." *Tennessee Libraries* 38 (Fall): 13-16.

Ways in which to boost the use of a Kurzweil reading machine are discussed.

Kazlauskas, D. W., S. T. Weaver, and W. R. Jones. 1987. "Kurzweil Reading Machine: A Study of Usage Patterns." *Journal of Academic Librarianship* 12 (January): 356-58.

A study of the use of Kurzweil reading machines at 26 academic libraries indicates that they are underutilized.

Lackey, G. H. 1982. "For More Reading: Large Print Books or the Visolett? *Education of the Visually Handicapped* 14 (Fall): 87-94.

The results of this statistically detailed study show that students whose eye conditions respond well to magnification read significantly more with the visolett than they do with large-print books. This might suggest to the librarian that a visolett or similar magnifying device should be made available in the library for use by visually impaired patrons.

Library Technology Reports. 1981. 17 (November/December): entire issue.

This issue of the journal is devoted to library equipment for disabled patrons. It includes addresses, prices, and detailed descriptions and evaluations of equipment for the blind, physically disabled, hearing impaired, and deaf. Although dated, this still provides one of the most comprehensive overviews available. It should be used as a starting point for determining the availability of special devices.

Lisson, P. 1987. "Large Print Placebo." *Canadian Library Journal* 44 (February): 5-6.

Lisson makes the point that a large group of citizens are visually impaired (not blind) but that they are ignored because the needs of the blind seem more urgent. It is indicated that large print is not the complete answer to the needs of visually impaired patrons because it is too expensive. Magnifiers and other sight enhancers that can be used with the less expensive regular print resources already available in a library are considered to be more beneficial.

Mandelstam, M. 1988. "Thesaurus on Equipment for Disabled People." *Journal of Documentation* 44 (June): 144-58.
A thesaurus of terms for use in electronic retrieval of information about assistive devices for disabled individuals is presented.

McCormick, E. 1990. "Volunteers to Produce Braille on Demand from Floppy Disks." *American Libraries* 21 (February): 99.
Through a method of storing the coding for braille on computer readable disks, a computer can be connected to a high-speed braille embosser that can produce a braille book in 20 to 30 minutes.

National Technical Information Service. 1987. *Computers for the Handicapped: January 1983-March 1987.* NTIS PB87-8562411.
This report provides guidance regarding computer systems designed for the handicapped. Systems discussed include braille keyboards and printers, translation systems that translate characters into braille sound activated keyboards, computers controlled by eye movements, and speech synthesizers. Computer bulletin boards for the visually handicapped and a mechanical hand used to communicate between a blind-deaf person and a computer are discussed. The 155 citations are fully indexed.

Weinberg, B. 1980. "The Kurzweil Machine: Half a Miracle." *American Libraries* 11 (November): 603-4, 627.
A research project at the New York Public Library suggests that the Kurzweil machine will fail to reach its potential audience of blind readers unless abundant library staff support is provided.

Willoughby, E. L. 1988. "Library Services in a School for the Blind." *Catholic Library World* 60 (November/December): 120-21.
The special formats and services provided blind patrons at the Overbrook School for the Blind include standard reference works in print and braille, AV material, a Kurzweil reading machine, a touch and learn center, a braille card catalog, and computer enhancements that produce enlarged screen output.

Attitudes

Attitudes toward Handicapped People, Past and Present. 1984. Washington, D.C.: National Library Service for the Blind and Physically Handicapped, Library of Congress.

    This annotated bibliography of books, periodical articles, films, and bibliographies about attitudes toward disabled persons is updated regularly by the National Library Service and is an excellent collection building resource.

Begg, R. 1979. "Disabled Libraries: An Examination of Physical and Attitudinal Barriers to Handicappped Library Users." *Law Library Journal* 72 (Summer): 513-25.

    Beginning with a brief summary of legislation pertaining to handicapped access, the author outlines professional responsibilities for accessibility as well as specifics of physical and attitudinal accessibility. Although old, the ethics espoused are still relevant and are beautifully stated.

Eldridge, L. 1982. *Speaking Out: Personal and Professional Views on Library Service for Blind and Physically Handicapped Individuals*. Washington, D.C.: National Library Service for the Blind and Physically Handicapped, Library of Congress.

    This compilation of interviews with librarians, students, educators, and users of library services for the blind and physically disabled focuses on the interviewees' feelings and experiences.

Bibliographic Instruction

Currie, M., and D. McLean-Howe. 1988. "Bibliographic Instruction for the Print Handicapped." *College and Research Library News* 49 (November): 672-74.

    Guidelines for providing bibliographic instruction to print handicapped individuals are provided.

Wesson, C. L., and M. Keefe. 1989. "Teaching Library Skills to Special Education Students." *School Library Media Quarterly* 17 (Winter): 71-77.

    Guidelines and procedures for assessing special education students' proficiency levels regarding library use and for planning and implementing library instruction are presented.

Bibliography

Baskin, B. H., and K. H. Harris. 1984. *More Notes from a Different Drummer.* New York: Bowker.

    This comprehensive annotated guide to juvenile fiction (written between 1976 and 1981) that depicts handicapped characters is considered a classic.

_____. 1977. *Notes from a Different Drummer.* New York: Bowker.

    This is a comprehensive annotated guide to juvenile fiction (written between 1940 and 1975) that depicts handicapped characters.

Bauman, M. K. 1976. *Blindness, Visual Impairment, Deafblindness: An Annotated Listing of the Literature, 1953-75.* Philadelphia, Pa: Temple University Press.

    This annotated bibliography of nonmedical, mostly monographic literature about blindness, visual impairment, and related topics is periodically updated in the journal *Blindness, Visual Impairment, Deaf Blindness: Semi-annual Listing of Current Literature.*

Bopp, R. E. 1980. "Periodicals for the Disabled: Their Importance as Information Sources." *Serials Librarian* 5 (Winter): 61-70.

    This annotated listing of periodical literature published by and/or for disabled persons is helpful for collection development. Although the article is old, the periodicals listed are for the most part still published and still considered core purchases.

_____. 1982. "Physically Disabled People, Personal Narratives: A Review of Recent Works." *Reference Services Review* 10 (Spring): 45-48.

    An annotated list of published personal narratives by physically disabled persons, this may be helpful for bibliotherapy applications.

_____. 1981. "Rehabilitation Literature: A Guide to Selection Materials." *Library Resources and Technical Services* 25 (July/September): 228-43.

    Bopp describes and evaluates various selection tools on the basis of their coverage of rehabilitation literature and their usefulness to academic, public, and special librarians. This is still useful, even with its older publication date.

Building a Library Collection on Blindness and Physical Handicaps: Basic Materials and Resources. 1989. Washington, D.C.: National Library Service for the Blind and Physically Handicapped, Library of Congress.

This listing contains materials recommended to libraries and organizations as basic resources for the provision of current information services on visual and physical disabilities. The list is divided by subject and is updated quarterly in the publication *Added Entries* (published by the Library of Congress National Library Service for the Blind and Physically Handicapped).

Craver, K. W. 1983. "Counseling the Handicapped: An Annotated Bibliography for Children, Counselors, and Parents." *Reference Services Review* 81 (Fall): 25-42.

This is very thorough and includes fiction, bibliographies, online bibliographic resources, nonfiction, audiovisual materials, and so on.

Crichton, J. 1989. "Travel Books for the Disabled." *Publisher's Weekly* 235 (20 January): 60.

Publications that provide information uniquely useful to disabled travelers are identified and discussed.

Dalton, P. I. 1986. "Periodical Resources on Deafness and Hearing Impairment." *Serials Librarian* 10 (Spring): 61-68.

Dalton discusses magazines and other periodicals such as journals, newsletters, and newspapers that deal with deafness and hearing impairment. Each magazine is described with an annotation that includes the characteristics of the publication and the audience it will attract. Sources are provided for other publications as well.

Friedburg, J. B., J. B. Mullins, and A. W. Sukiennik. 1985. *Accept Me as I Am*. New York: Bowker.

This annotated guide to juvenile nonfiction about disabilities selectively lists recommended nonfiction within disability group categories.

Hirschberg, R. 1982. "The Developmentally Disabled in Literature for Young People." *Catholic Library World* 53, no. 9: 391-94.

The author provides selection criteria by which to judge materials that portray developmentally disabled individuals. She then evaluates several titles in terms of the selection criteria as models of ways in which to apply the criteria.

Lande, H. 1953. *Books about the Blind: A Bibliographic Guide to Literature Relating to the Blind*. New York: The William Byrd Press.

One of the first attempts to list nonmedical literature related to visual impairment, this has historical value and is considered a classic in the field.

LiBretto, E. V., ed. 1990. *High-Low Handbook: Books, Materials, and Services for the Problem Reader*. 3d ed. New York: Bowker.
    Like the second edition (1985), this invaluable resource describes high/low readers, provides information on how to evaluate high/low reading material, and provides an annotated listing of a recommended core of high/low reading materials.

Mellon, C. A. 1989. "Evaluating the Portrayal of Disabled Characters in Juvenile Fiction." *Journal of Youth Services in Libraries* 2 (Winter): 143-50.
    As he narrates personal experiences with reading, the author discusses the need to portray disabled characters in literature realistically.

_____. 1989. "Exceptionality in Children's Books: Combining Apples and Oranges." *School Library Journal* 35 (October): 46-47.
    This article discusses the great need for books on a wide range of disabilities that stress the similarities rather than the differences between disabled and nondisabled children.

Velleman, R. A. 1980. "Library Service to the Disabled: An Annotated Bibliography of Journals and Newsletters." *Serials Librarian* 5 (Winter): 49-60.
    This bibliography offers a basic listing of journals in the fields of medical and vocational rehabilitation and special education. It also lists journals written for disabled persons themselves. The continuing need for a central clearinghouse is cited. Much of the information here is still useful, although it has been updated in Velleman's monograph (listed under the general category in this bibliography).

Weber, D. J. 1981. "Periodicals Supporting Library Service for the Blind and Physically Handicapped." *Serials Review* 7 (April/June): 45-47.
    This annotated list of primary print periodicals published in support of library service for the physically disabled is older but still accurate.

Bibliotherapy

Elser, H. 1982. Bibliotherapy in Practice." *Library Trends* 30, no. 4 (Spring): 647-59.

The author's experience with adolescents in a bibliotherapy group is discussed. The author suggests that the best approach upon which to initiate discussions is music, including song lyrics and biographies of performers. Other methods suggested are the use of psychodrama and role reversal.

Rubin, R. J. 1978. *Bibliotherapy Sourcebook*. Phoenix: Oryx Press.

This anthology of articles on bibliotherapy contains selections from librarians, educators, medical professionals, and social service professionals. It is an excellent complement to Rubin's overview (*Using Bibliotherapy*), going into more detail and covering a broader range of bibliotherapeutic topics.

_____. 1978. *Using Bibliotherapy: A Guide to Theory and Practice*. Phoenix: Oryx Press.

The history of bibliotherapy is discussed, the theories and approaches are enumerated, its relation to librarianship is considered, and training recommendations are given. Bibliographies of appropriate juvenile and adult reading materials are included.

Blindness/Visual Impairment

Arditi, A., and A. E. Gillman. 1986. "Computing for the Blind User." *Byte* 11 (March): 199-200, 202, 204, 206, 208.

The author examines some of the problems that blind users face in using computers. Problems include poorly designed speech synthesizers, difficulties proofreading text spoken by a synthesizer, and complicated keyboards. Designing hardware and software from the "bottom up" rather than adapting existing equipment is advocated.

Brugsch, H. 1986. "Braille-Edit." *Byte* 11 (March): 251-52, 254, 256, 258.

Braille-Edit is a talking word processor for the visually impaired. The program works with Apple computers and allows users to hear menus with the use of a speech synthesizer. It also allows proofreading of text by hearing it spoken.

Eldridge, L. 1985. *R Is for Reading: Library Service to Blind and Physically Handicapped Children*. National Library Service for the Blind and Physically Handicapped, Library of Congress.

This contains interviews with parents, counselors, reading specialists, and librarians regarding their uses of, and suggestions for improvements of, the National Library Service for the Blind and Physically Handicapped.

Hagle, A. D. "Information Access by Blind and Physically Handicapped Persons." In *Advances in Librarianship*, edited by Wesley Simonton, vol. 3, 247-75. New York: Academic Press, 1982.

This interesting article provides definitions and statistics concerning persons with visual and physical disabilities in the United States, lists and gives addresses of agencies that provide special library services and resources, and has sections on braille electronic reading machines, paperless braille, optacon machines, braille computer terminals, voice synthesizers, speech compression, voice indexing of audiocassettes, computer-assisted lipreading for the deaf, bibliographic control of special materials, and international cooperation.

Havens, S. 1987. "Large Print in Focus." *Library Journal* 112 (July): 32-34.

Havens discusses large-print books in public libraries in terms of funding, purchasing, the library population that uses these materials, and library services and outreach programs.

Lauer, H. L. 1989. "Why One Medium Isn't Enough." *OCLC Micro* 5 (December): 22-25.

The author justifies the need for braille, audiotapes, talking computers, and paperless braille.

Michaels, C. L. "Our Ears as Channels of Information." In *Library Literacy Means Lifelong Learning*, edited by Carolyn Leopold Michaels, 149-170. Metuchen, N.J.: Scarecrow Press, 1985.

The author discusses educators' use of multimedia packages, tapes, records, radios, and videotapes to bring content to special groups.

National Library Service for the Blind and Physically Handicapped. 1983. *That All May Read: Library Services for the Blind and Physically Handicapped*. Washington, D.C.: Library of Congress.

This provides an overview of the needs of individuals unable to use print resources and describes current and historic services and practices designed to meet these needs.

Shaw, A. E. 1986. "Better Services for the Visually Handicapped." *Library Association Record* 88 (February): 85.

Blind and partially sighted speakers enumerate their needs: that librarians recognize their role as key in providing access to the range of information available in recorded formats; that magnifiers and appropriate lighting are significant aids; that library signs written in large, clear print are critical; and that high-tech equipment is often helpful. Also emphasized is the importance of outreach programs.

Storm, M., ed. 1977. *Library Service to the Blind and Physically Handicapped.* Metuchen, N.J.: Scarecrow Press.

This compilation of journal articles focuses on the reading needs of visually and physically disabled persons.

What Do You Do When You See a Blind Person? 1980. Presented by the American Foundation for the Blind. Produced and edited by Si Fried. Written and directed by Arthur Zigouras. New Brunswick, N.J.: Phoenix Films.

Although old, this videotape still makes its point through humorous interactions between a blind man and a sighted man.

White, E. C. 1985. "Library Service to the Blind: Progress through Technology and Social Awareness." *Catholic Library World* 56 (May): 434-37.

This provides a history of library services available to the blind, with emphasis on progress owing to technological advances.

Catalogs and Directories

Catalog of Captioned Films/Videos for the Deaf. 1989-1990. Prepared by the Modern Talking Picture Service, Inc., Washington, D.C.: Captioning and Adaptation Branch. Office of Special Education and Rehabilitative Services, U.S. Department of Education. Updates issued periodically.

This listing of available captioned films includes film synopses, running time, and ratings.

Complete Directory of Large Print Books and Serials. Published annually. New York: Bowker.

Produced in large-print format, this includes general reading materials, textbooks, newspapers, and periodicals that have been produced in 14-point or larger type. Entries give the same information about the books as that provided in *Books in Print*, but the resource lists many titles that are not included in *Books in Print*.

Directory of Radio Reading Services Offering Programming for Persons with Limitations in Reading Print. Published annually. New York: American Foundation for the Blind in cooperation with the Association of Radio Reading Services. Tampa, Fla.: Association of Radio Reading Services.

    The directory provides addresses, phone numbers, and services offered by Radio Reading Services throughout the country.

Magazines in Special Media. 1989. Washington, D.C.: National Library Service for the Blind and Physically Handicapped, Library of Congress.

    This lists over 300 magazine titles in various formats (recorded and braille), which can be obtained through direct circulation, direct loan, or interlibrary loan from the NLS or through paid subscriptions.

Recording for the Blind Catalog of Recorded Books. 1990. New York: Recording for the Blind. Supplements are published periodically.

    This is a useful catalog of the over 72,000 books recorded by Recording for the Blind and available to eligible blind and visually impaired persons.

Redmond, L., comp. 1987. *Reading Materials in Large Type*. Washington, D.C.: National Library Service for the Blind and Physically Handicapped, Library of Congress.

    This catalog, when used in combination with the *Complete Directory of Large Print Books and Serials* (see listing in this section of the bibliography), provides almost total coverage of large-print publication.

_____. 1983. *Reading, Writing, and Other Communication Aids for Visually and Physically Handicapped Persons*. Washington, D.C.: National Library Service for the Blind and Physically Handicapped, Library of Congress.

    This listing of products includes descriptions of the devices as well as prices and addresses of the companies from which they may be obtained. Company addresses are for the most part still accurate (as of 1990), but prices will have to be doublechecked.

Deafness and Hearing Impairment

American Library Association. Association of Specialized and Cooperative Library Agencies. Standards for Library Service to the Deaf Subcommittee. 1981. "Techniques for Library Service to the Deaf and Hard of Hearing." *Interface* 4 (Fall): 2-3.
>The committee provides guidance to all types of libraries in the areas of communications, resources, publicity, programs, and staffing.

Dalton, P. I. 1985. *Library Service to the Deaf and Hearing Impaired*. Phoenix: Oryx Press.
>This is the definitive full-length resource on library services for deaf patrons. It is essential for library professional collections.

"The Deaf." 1980. *Interface* 3 (Fall): 6-8.
>A brief profile of the deaf population is given. Also presented are short discussions on captioned television in the library and the value of the *Red Notebook*.

Duke, D. 1986. "The Librarian's Role in Fulfilling the Needs of the Hearing-Impaired Child." *Kentucky Libraries* 50 (Summer): 3-4, 6-8.
>This concise summary of the effects of deafness on language development, reading skills, and communication includes specific suggestions for teaching library skills to hearing impaired students.

Esteves, R. 1982. "Video Opens Libraries to the Deaf: New Visual Techniques Show How Poorly Printed Materials Serve the Clientele." *American Libraries* 13 (January): 36, 38.
>The author presents recommendations and examples of how closed-captioning, signed programs, and color video cameras can be used to expand the library's accessibility to deaf patrons.

Freese, M. 1986. "Library Service for Deaf and Hard-of-Hearing Individuals." *Illinois Libraries* 68 (November): entire issue.
>This very helpful issue includes general suggestions of services as well as listings of special agencies, publishers, assistive devices for hearing impaired people, and high interest/low vocabulary materials.

Hagemeyer, A. 1975. *Deaf Awareness Handbook for Public Librarians*. Washington, D.C.: Public Library of the District of Columbia.
>Although this document is old, much of the information is still applicable to all types of libraries. It includes definitions of deafness;

sections on communication techniques, materials, and resources; and suggestions of special library services for the deaf.

———. 1982. "Library Service and Outreach Programs for the Deaf." *Wyoming Library Roundup* 38 (Fall): 15-21; also in *Illinois Libraries* 63 (September 1981): 530-34.

This is a transcription of a speech in which the author (a deaf librarian) emphasizes service to deaf and hearing impaired patrons via the librarian's attitudes toward deafness and their awareness of the resources (such as the *Red Notebook*) available to deaf patrons.

Kretschmer, R. E. 1981. "Living with a Hearing Impairment." *Illinois Libraries* 63 (September): 515-20.

The author presents information on how hearing impairments affect the manner in which an individual develops and functions in society.

Lawton, B. 1989. "Library Instruction Needs Assessment: Designing Survey Instruments." *Research Strategies* 7 (Summer): 119-28.

Surveys used to determine the library instruction needs of deaf and hearing impaired patrons are presented and their efficacy discussed.

Lewis, P. 1988. "Breaking Silence – Reaching Out to Persons Who Are Deaf and Hearing Impaired." *Bookmark* 46 (Summer): 252-55.

Library services to the deaf at the Queens Borough Public Library include TDD service, materials on deafness and signing, captioned films, assistive devices, individualized service, literacy programs, sign language instruction, and programs that reflect the input of deaf members on the library's programming committee.

Low, K. 1989. "Telecommunications Devices for the Deaf." *American Libraries* 20 (May): 446.

This is a listing of TDDs available from two prominent manufacturers (Krown Research and Ultratech). The listings include prices and specifications on the machines.

Metcalf, M. J. 1981. "Library Services for the Hearing Impaired." *Illinois Libraries* 63 (October): 626-33.

Problems of hearing impaired individuals are detailed, and model programs of service in public libraries are outlined.

Modica, M. 1987/1988. "The Captioned Film/Video Program for the Deaf." *Sightlines* 21 (Winter): 6-7.

Ways of evaluating whether a film can successfully be closed-captioned, as well as the procedures and intellectual processes of closed-captioning are described.

Monroe, J. 1986. "Focus on Youth: Improving Services to the Deaf." *Collection Building* 8 no. 3:37-40.

Practical suggestions concerning collection development for deaf patrons and techniques for effective communication are presented.

Mulaiski, C. 1987. "Academic Library Service to Deaf Students: Survey and Recommendations." *RQ* 26 (Summer): 477-86.

A survey yields recommendations to improve reference service to handicapped college students. Among the suggestions are more outreach, inservice education for staff, and more regular contact and cooperation between staff and students.

Prine, S., and K. Wright. 1982. "Standards for the Visually and Hearing Impaired." *Library Trends* 31 (Summer): 93-108.

Prine and Wright provide a succinct historical summary of the ALA standards for library service to the blind and visually impaired. Standards for service to the hearing impaired are also mentioned.

Sangster, C. 1986. "Guidelines for Library Service to Hearing Impaired Persons." *Bookmark* 44 (Winter): 104-8.

The formats of materials most suitable for hearing impaired readers (print and nonprint) are discussed.

Vesely, M., and S. Galloway. 1988. "Library Service to Hearing Impaired People." *Bookmark* 46 (Summer): 255-56.

This checklist for implementing appropriate library services for the deaf covers library accessibility, staff awareness, special services, programs, activities, and equipment.

Education of Librarians

Karp, R. S. 1987. "Library Services to Disabled Individuals and Library School Curricula." *Interface* 9, no. 4 (Summer): 9-10.

Karp describes the content of a course on library services to disabled individuals and emphasizes the need for such services to be considered as a necessary part of a library school's core curriculum.

Wright, K. C. 1987. "Educating Librarians about Service to Special Groups: The Emergence of Disabled Persons into the Mainstream." *North Carolina Libraries* 45 (Summer): 79-82.

Wright discusses ways in which library schools and inservice workshops can teach about library services to disabled patrons.

General

American Library Association. 1988. "Resolution on Access to the Use of Libraries and Information by Individuals with Physical or Mental Impairments." In *Intellectual Freedom Manual*, 113-14. Chicago: American Library Association.

Adopted by the American Library Association on 13 January 1988, the ALA statement clearly spells out that the "Library Bill of Rights" ensures access for and prohibits discrimination against individuals with physical or mental impairments.

Association on Handicapped Student Service Programs in Post Secondary Education. 1988. *AHSSPPE Inservice Education Kit*. Columbus, Ohio: Association on Handicapped Student Service Programs in Post Secondary Education.

This excellent multimedia resource provides a taped two-hour lecture on disabilities (mobility, visual, hearing, and learning) and their remediation in a classroom setting. Handouts, exercises, and audiovisual materials are included in the packet.

Baskin, B. H., and K. H. Harris. 1982. *The Mainstreamed Library: Issues, Ideas, Innovations*. Chicago: American Library Association.

This compilation of articles focuses on the issues that librarians must confront to meet the challenges posed by mainstreaming, changes in policies and practices that must be made, and the ways in which traditional services can be modified, broadened, or replaced to meet the special needs of this population. The volume includes discussions of physical accessibility, materials selection, and outreach programs.

Dequin, H. C. 1983. *Librarians Serving Disabled Children and Young People*. Littleton, Colo.: Libraries Unlimited.

This general reference emphasizes the services that public and school librarians can provide for disabled patrons from kindergarten through high school. Especially helpful is its inclusion of selection criteria for special materials.

Green, Kerry. 1980. "Services for the Handicapped." *Media and Methods* 16 (March): 39-40. ERIC Doc. No. EJ 217 595.

Ways in which AV personnel can meet the needs of disabled students by analyzing their needs, matching the needs with services, improving staff awareness, conducting publicity, and keeping records are suggested in a concise manner.

Howard, Cate. 1984. "Exceptional Children: How Do We Serve Them?" *North Carolina Libraries* 42 (Fall): 127-28.

Howard discusses ways in which to accommodate disabled children during storytime and other children's programming. A short list of libraryoriented books on this topic is given.

Karrenbrock, M. H., and L. Lucas. 1986. "Libraries and Disabled Persons: A Review of Selected Research." In *Advances in Library Administration and Organization*, vol. 6, 241-306. Greenwich, Ct.: JAI Press.

This report of research conducted since 1903 provides a starting point for administrators interested in planning programs for disabled persons and for researchers planning future study.

Lang, J., ed. 1988. *Unequal Access to Information Resources: Problems and Needs of the World's Information Poor*. Ann Arbor, Mich.: Pierian Press.

The sixth chapter of this excellent monograph has articles by Wright and Davie (detailing the discrimination that disabled people suffer), Dalton (presenting a model for library services for the deaf), Huang (providing information about assistive devices and federal legislation for disabled people), and Dequin (presenting the results of a survey of 442 librarians regarding their attitudes toward disabled people).

Lucas, L., and M. H. Karrenbrock. 1983. *The Disabled Child in the Library*. Littleton, Colo.: Libraries Unlimited.

Similar to Dequin's (see listing under general category in the bibliography) resource, this also focuses on library services to disabled children. However, unlike Dequin, Lucas and Karrenbrock take a disability approach, dividing information into sections by disability. Especially helpful is the selection criteria chart in the appendix.

Rovenger, J. 1987. "Learning Differences/Library Directions: Library Service to Children with Learning Differences." *Library Trends* 35 (Winter): 427-35.

Rovenger provides some interesting sensitizing activities and discusses accommodations that librarians can make for learning disabled, hearing impaired, and visually impaired young patrons.

Ryder, J., ed. 1987. *Library Services to Housebound People: A Practical Guide*. London: Library Association.
This book provides suggestions regarding the provision of library services to the housebound. The final chapter examines services such as community information, large-print books, circulation of tapes, reading aids, and services to institutionalized handicapped.

Thomas, J. L. 1980. *Meeting the Needs of the Handicapped: A Resource for Teachers and Librarians*. Phoenix: Oryx Press.
This group of articles selected from educational journals published between 1973 and 1979 addresses many different disabilities and offers suggestions for appropriate programs and activities.

Thomas, J. L., and C. H. Thomas. 1982. *Library Services for the Handicapped Adult*. Phoenix: Oryx Press.
In an extremely clear and interesting format, the Thomases have gathered essays that deal with different aspects of services for disabled adults. This is not an overview, but an idea starter.

Velleman, R. A. 1990. *Meeting the Needs of People with Disabilities: A Guide for Librarians, Educators, and Other Service Professionals*. Phoenix: Oryx Press.
Primarily focused on physical disabilities, this provides definitions, consumer information, rehabilitation and special education information, and information for librarians on a vast array of topics.

Watson, E. S. 1984. "Model Disability Awareness Day." *Interracial Books for Children Bulletin* 15, no. 3: 11-13, 22.
This delightful and informative account of one elementary school's disability awareness day program includes a step-by-step description of how the project was planned as well as lists of sources (names and addresses) of free or low-cost materials, speakers, and recommended books.

Wright, K. C., and J. F. Davie. 1989. *Library and Information Services for Handicapped Individuals*. 3d ed. Englewood, Colo.: Libraries Unlimited.

Now in its third edition, this general resource describes major disabled groups and suggests general accommodations. Attitudinal accessibility is emphasized.

Learning Disabilities

ACB's [*sic*] *of Learning Disabilities*. 1987. Produced by Carolyn Trice. Directed by Ken Morrison. New Orleans: The Film Company.
   This videotape presents sensitizing activities and information about different types of learning disabilities. It is quite comprehensive and very helpful.

Ahlen, B. 1989. "The Library and Dyslexics." *Scandinavian Public Library Quarterly* 22, no. 2: 18-20.
   The role of the library in providing talking books/print books combinations for learning disabled patrons is discussed. The need for flexible loan periods is also emphasized.

Blankenship, M. E., J. E. Lokerson, and K. A. Verbeke. 1989. "Folk and Fairy Tales for the Learning Disabled: Tips for Enhancing Understanding and Enjoyment." *School Library Media Quarterly* 17 (Summer): 200-205.
   Academic and social behaviors typical of learning disabled students are described and ideas for developing and modifying lessons are presented. Characteristics of folk and fairy tales, which offer valuable literary opportunities but present special difficulties for learning disabled students, are discussed, and methods for helping students deal with the characteristics are presented.

Bliss, B. A. 1986. "Dyslexics as Library Users." *Library Trends* 35 (Fall): 293-302.
   Characteristics of dyslexic library users are discussed, as are suggestions for accommodating their special needs.

Bloom, J. 1990. *Help Me to Help My Child: A Sourcebook for Parents of Learning Disabled Children*. Boston: Little, Brown and Co.
   As the parents of children with learning disabilities search for answers and guidance in a variety of texts, they often become just as frustrated as their children. Bloom emphasizes that because there is no single cause for all learning disorders, there is no single solution. She attempts not to find a solution but rather to provide a vast array of information that parents must have to take charge of getting the help their children need.

Bryan, T. H., and J. H. Bryan. 1986. *Understanding Learning Disabilities*. Palo Alto, Calif.: Mayfield Publishing.

This comprehensive text provides detailed technical information about learning disabilities, their diagnosis, and ways to accommodate them. Although directed at teachers, it is an invaluable informational resource for librarians and parents.

Hammill, D. D. 1990. "On Defining Learning Disabilities: An Emerging Consensus." *Journal of Learning Disabilities* 23, no. 2 (February): 74-85.

Definitions of learning disability are traced historically from 1962 to the present.

Rovenger, J. 1984. "Library Services to Children with Learning Disabilities." *Bookmark* 43 (Fall): 27-30.

Rovenger discusses methods of adapting library services to children with learning disabilities and other special needs children. She emphasizes the importance of storytelling and stresses that there is a connection between written and oral language and learning to read.

Sawyer, G. 1989. "Sitting on the Bean Bags: Developing a Library for Children with Learning Difficulties." *School Libraries* 37 (May): 46-47.

Suggestions of ways in which to integrate services for all students with learning disabilities are made. It is recognized that older students enjoy looking through picture books and recognizing the book characters as old friends.

Silver, L. B. 1988. *The Misunderstood Child: A Guide for Parents of Learning Disabled Children*. New York: McGraw Hill.

This excellent introduction to the field of learning disabilities provides very helpful definitions and descriptions of how learning disabilities manifest themselves, the most common diagnosis techniques, intervention techniques that can be used by parents and educators, and medical intervention techniques. This is a good addition to the library's collection on disabilities and is helpful professional reading as well.

Zola, M. 1985. "New Wine for Old Bottles: Picture Books for the Adolescent Reader." In *Adolescents, Literature, and Work with Youth*, edited by J.P. Weiner and R. M. Stein, 19-25. New York: Haworth Press.

Picture books suitable for adolescents are described in terms of categories (i.e., those that teach or inform; those that foster critical thinking skills) and are then recommended as alternatives to traditional print resources. Although the disabled are not mentioned here in detail, the suggestions are easily applicable to learning disabled and mentally retarded adolescents.

Mental Retardation

Ark, C. E., and D. Charves. 1987. "Library Skills for DH Students in the Middle School." *Ohio Media Spectrum* 39 (Fall): 46-51.
    A schedule of library instruction for mentally retarded students in school is described.

Bird, W. 1985. "Computer Project at Western Carolina Center Library." *North Carolina Libraries* 43 (Fall): 164-65.
    At this center for the mentally retarded, microcomputers are successfully used to expand the use of leisure activity on the part of the residents.

Hodges, L. J. 1987. *Library Services for Persons Who Are Mentally Retarded: Guidelines*. Tallahassee: Florida Department of State, Division of Library and Information Services.
    This excellent and practical resource provides guidelines for working with mentally retarded patrons, their parents, and staff in institutions. Suggestions for programming are included.

_____. 1989. "You've Got What It Takes: Public Library Services to Persons Who Are Mentally Retarded." *RQ* 28 (Summer): 463-69.
    Hodges addresses attitudes of librarians toward mentally retarded patrons and makes concrete suggestions regarding services, collection development, and program planning for mentally retarded patrons.

Lucas, L. 1982. *Library Services to Developmentally Disabled Children and Adults*. Chicago: American Library Association.
    Services to retarded and nonretarded developmentally disabled individuals are outlined for public and school librarians.

Newberry, W. F. 1980. "The Last Unserved: Are Public Libraries Ready to Mainstream Mentally Retarded Patrons?" *American Libraries* 11: 218-20.
    The library behavior patterns of mentally retarded patrons are described, and questions about appropriate library services are asked.

Swensen, S. H. 1987. "Kim Can Also Read: A Picture Experience." *Bookbird* 25, no. 4 (December): 10-12.
    Swenson describes how textless picture books can allow mentally retarded children to "read" as they tell the story of the pictures.

Name/Subject Index